INTRODUCTION

This booklet contains over 40 recipes to provide new and seasoned members with fun easy recipes to support the body systems. There are recipes for roll-ons, sprays, scrubs, bath salts, and drinks. We hope to inspire people to use their starter kit essential oils and explore additional essential oils too.

Oily Yours,

Chelsa Bruno & Dana Ripepe

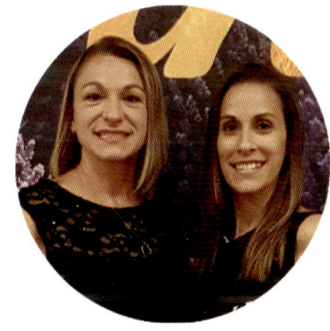

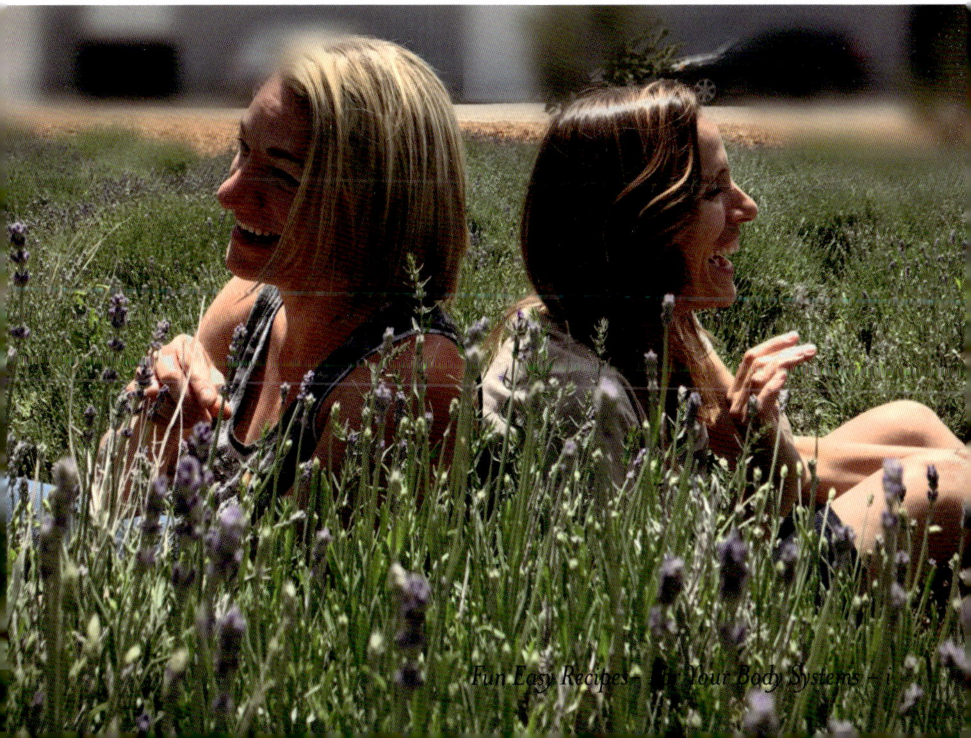

TABLE OF CONTENTS

Cardiovascular System Recipes 2-7

Digestive System Recipes 8-13

Endocrine System Recipes 14-19

Immune System Recipes 20-25

Integumentary System Recipes 26-31

Lymphatic System Recipes 32-37

Muscular/Skeletal System Recipes 38-43

Nervous System Recipes 44-49

Reproductive System: Women Recipes 50-55

Reproductive System: Men Recipes 56-61

Respiratory System Recipes 62-67

Urinary System Recipes 68-73

Fun Easy Recipes– For Your Body Systems – 1

CARDIOVASCULAR SYSTEM

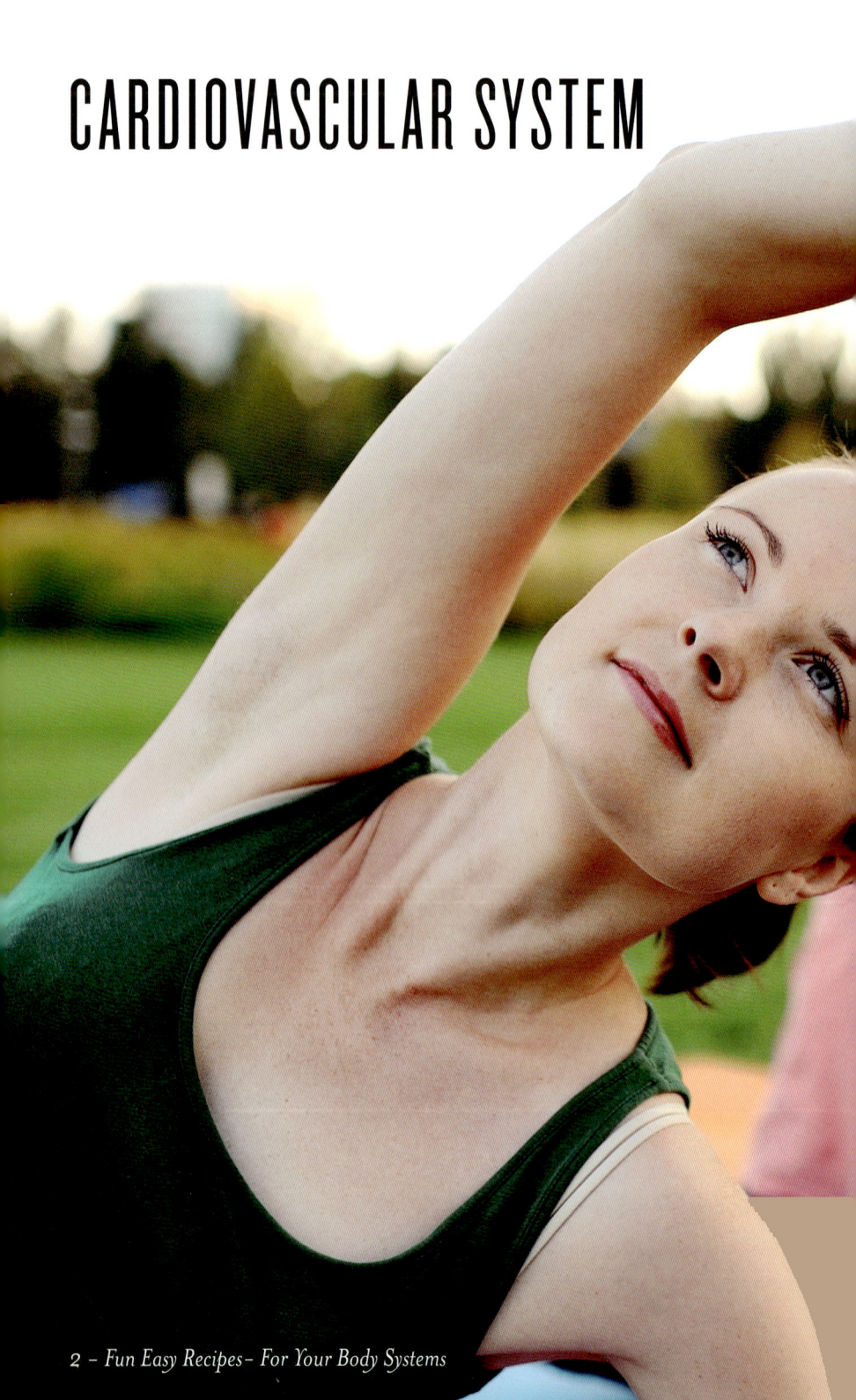

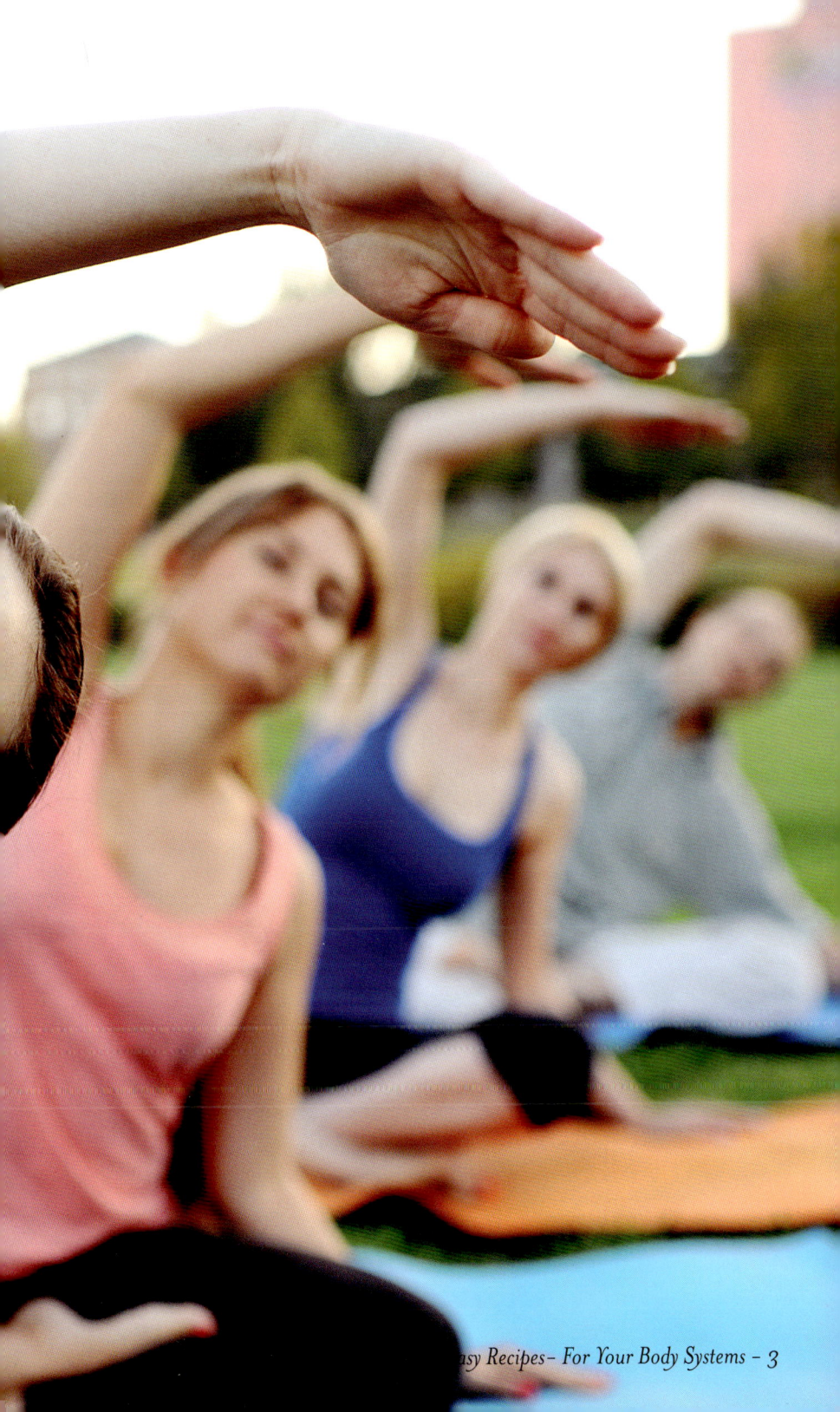

CARDIOVASCULAR SYSTEM

Roll-On

Ingredients:
- 10 drops AromaLife Essential Oil
- 5 drops Ylang Ylang Essential Oil
- V-6 Vegetable Oil
  (or Liquid Coconut Oil)
- 10 mL Glass Roll-On Bottle

Directions:
1. Add the Essential Oils into the roll-on bottle
2. Fill with V-6 Vegetable Oil and put on the roll-on top
3. Apply onto your wrists and chest to support the cardiovascular system

Bath Salts

Ingredients:
- 3 drops Stress Away Essential Oil
- 3 drops Peace & Calming Essential Oil
- 1/3 cup Epsom Salt
- 4 oz Glass Mason Jar

Directions:
1. Put the Epsom Salt, Stress Away and Peace & Calming Essential Oils into a glass bowl
2. Mix the ingredients together and place the mixture into the jar
3. Add 1 tablespoon of the mixture into your bath water to support the cardiovascular system

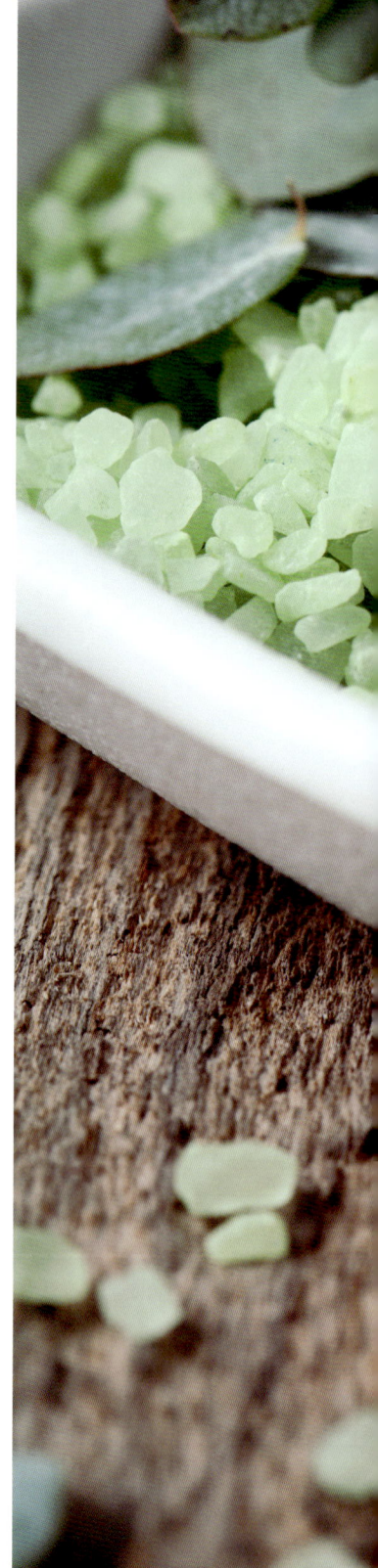

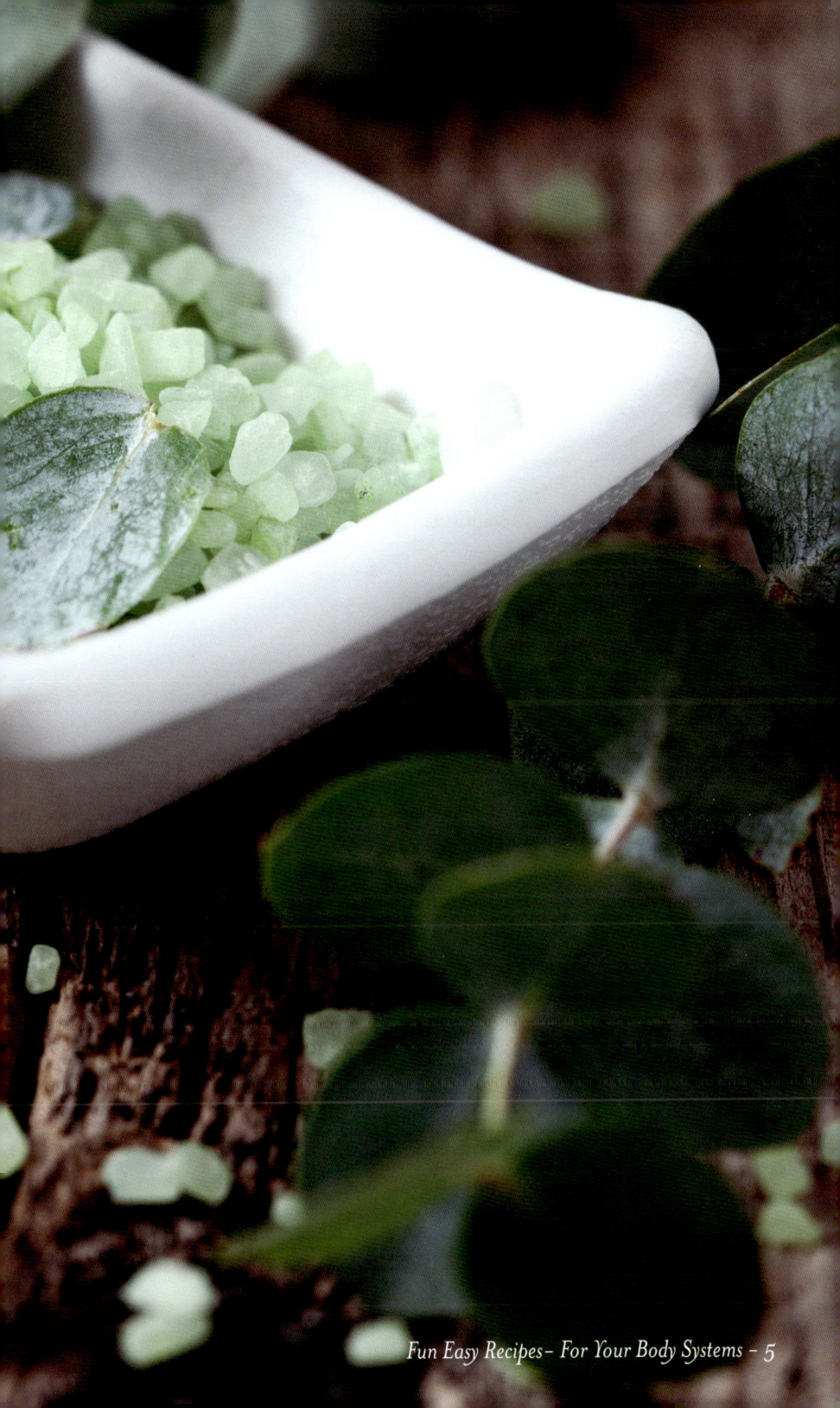

CARDIOVASCULAR SYSTEM

Diffuser Blend

Ingredients:
- 3 drops Peace & Calming Essential Oil
- 2 drops Ylang Ylang Essential Oil
- Water
- Diffuser

Directions:
1. Add water to the fill line of the diffuser
2. Put Peace & Calming and Ylang Ylang Essential Oils into the water
3. Put the top of the diffuser on and press the on button
4. Breathe in and relax.

Capsule

Ingredients:
- 4 drops Clove Vitality Essential Oil
- 4 drops Lemongrass Vitality Essential Oil
- Vegetable Capsule

Directions:
1. Add the Essential Oils into the capsule
2. Ingest one capsule for cardiovascular support as needed

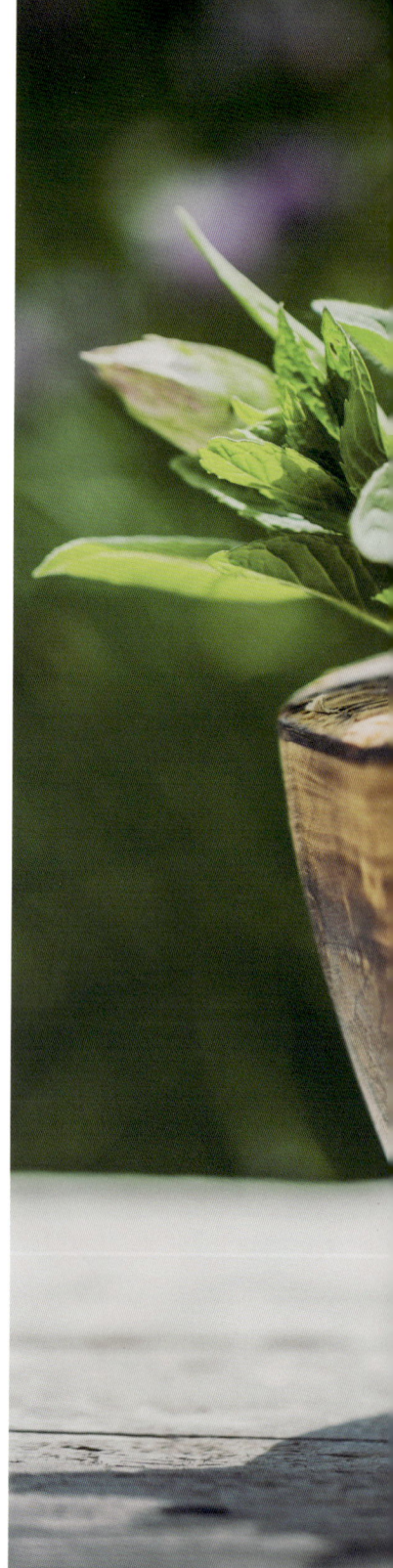

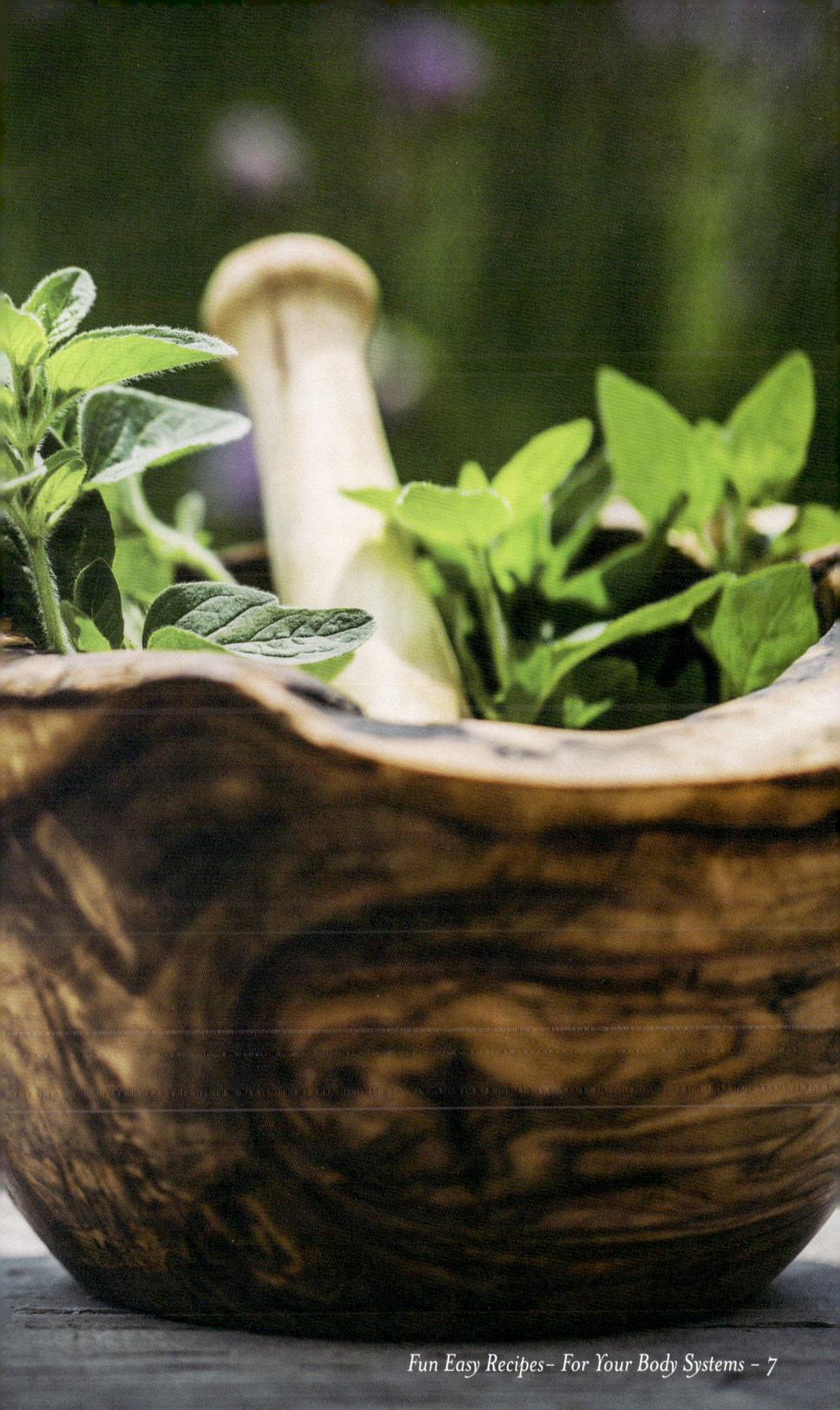

Fun Easy Recipes- For Your Body Systems - 7

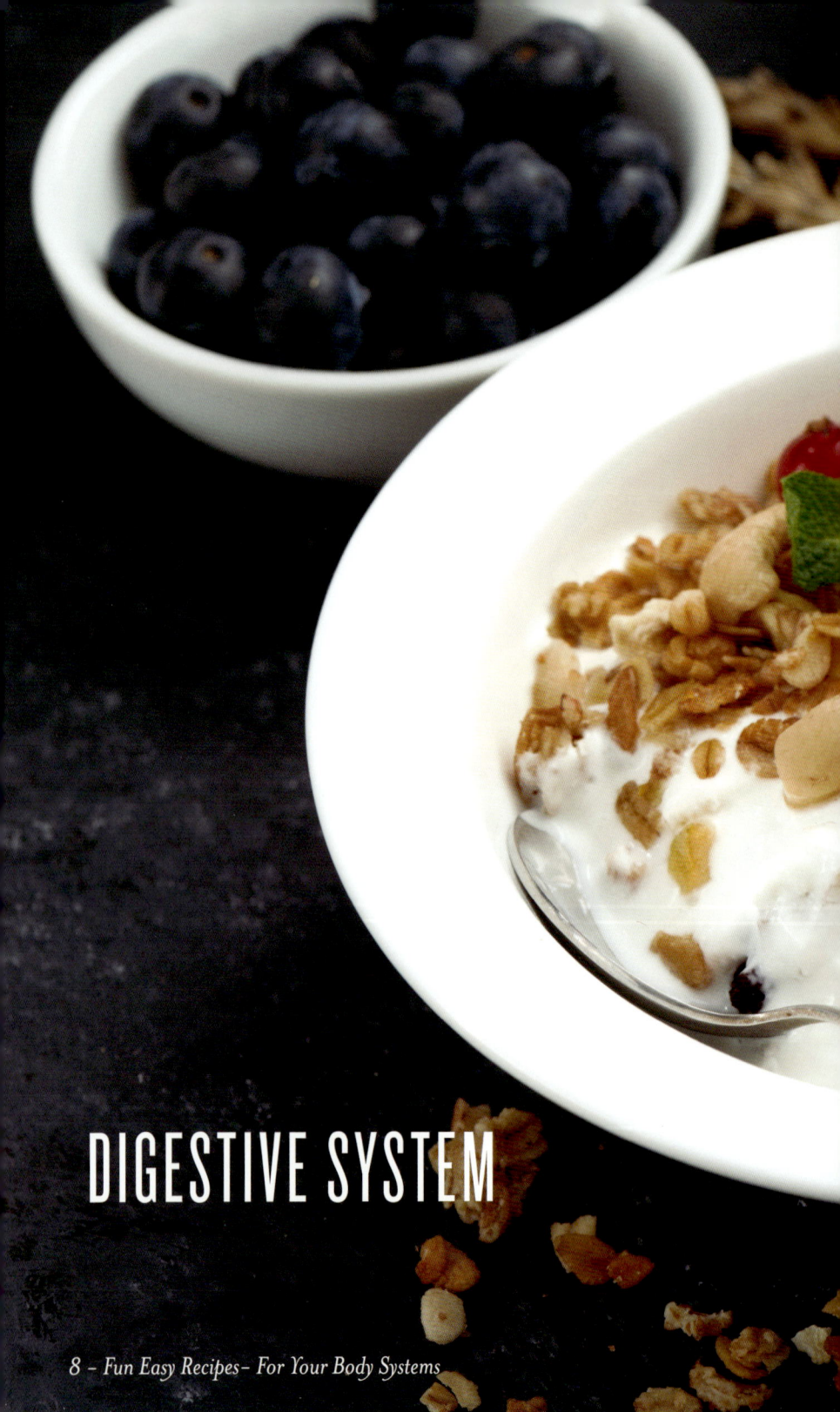

DIGESTIVE SYSTEM

8 – Fun Easy Recipes – For Your Body Systems

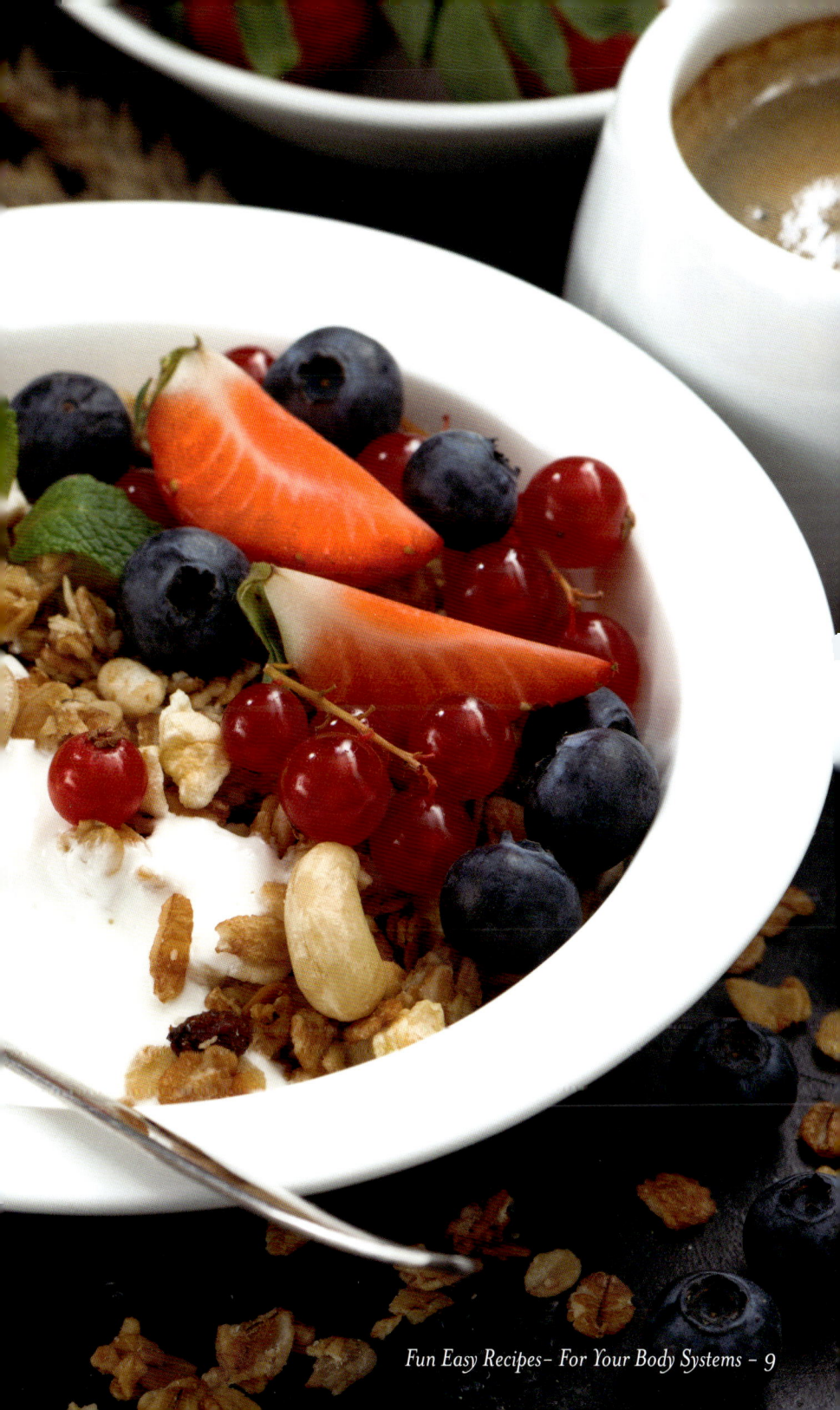

Fun Easy Recipes- For Your Body Systems - 9

DIGESTIVE SYSTEM

Roll-on

Ingredients:
- 6 drops Ginger Essential Oil
- 4 drops Fennel Essential Oil
- V-6 Vegetable Oil (or Liquid Coconut Oil)
- 10 mL Glass Roll-On Bottle

Directions:
1. Add the Essential Oils into the roll-on bottle
2. Fill with V-6 Vegetable Oil and put on the roll-on top
3. Apply onto your stomach to support the digestive system

Capsule

Ingredients:
- 4 drops DiGize Vitality Essential Oil
- 4 drops Peppermint Vitality Essential Oil
- Vegetable Capsule

Directions:
1. Add the Essential Oils into the capsule
2. Ingest one capsule for digestive support as needed

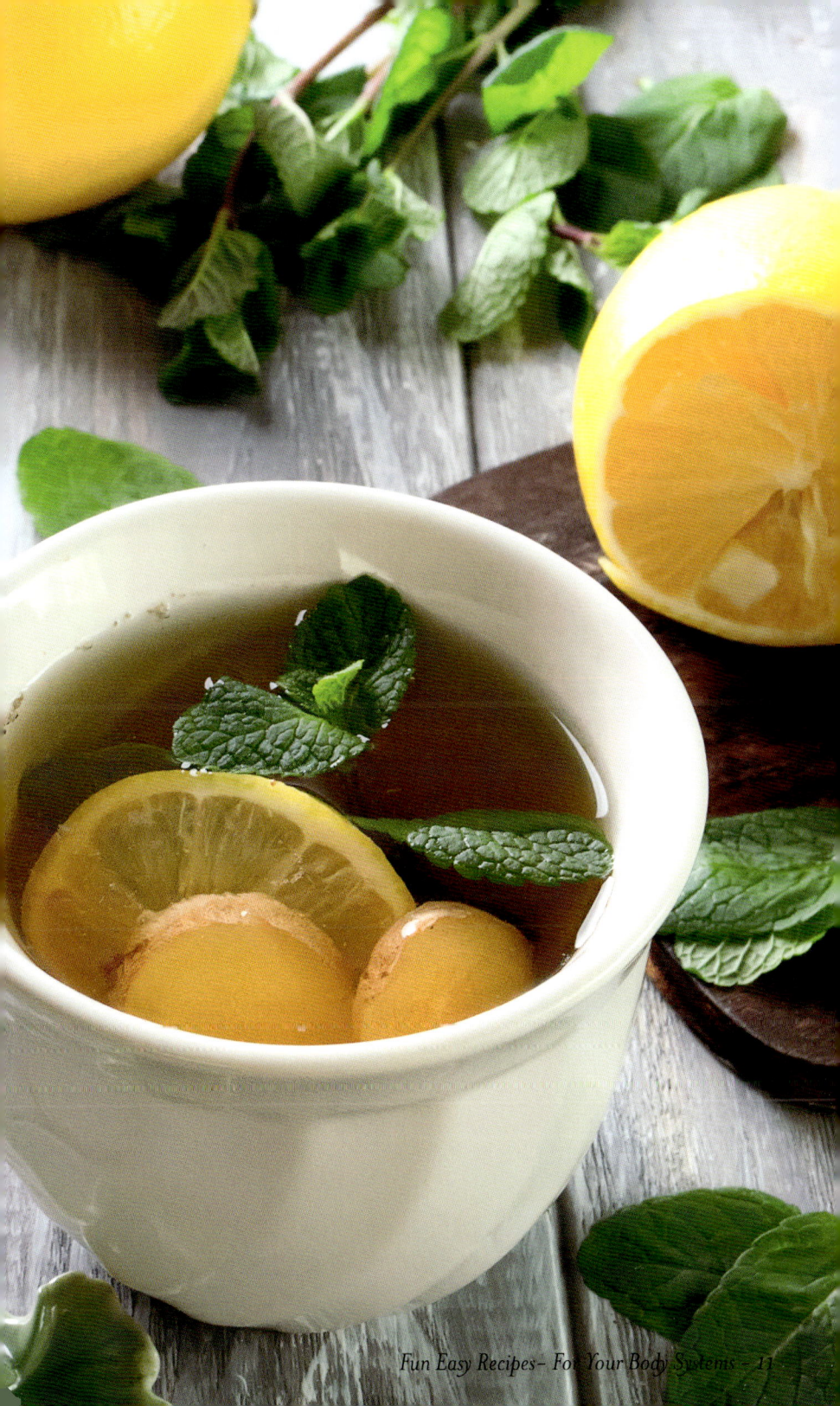

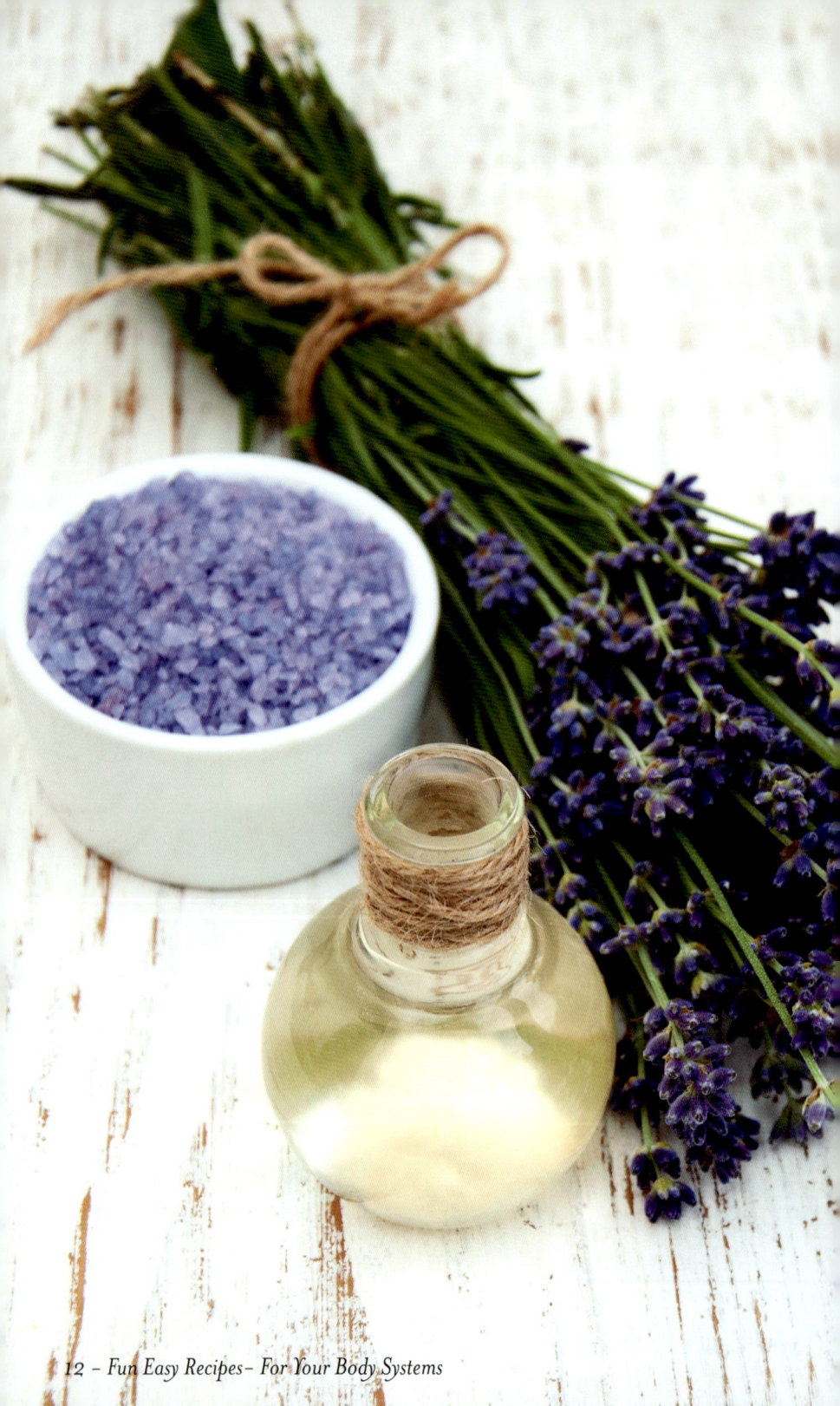

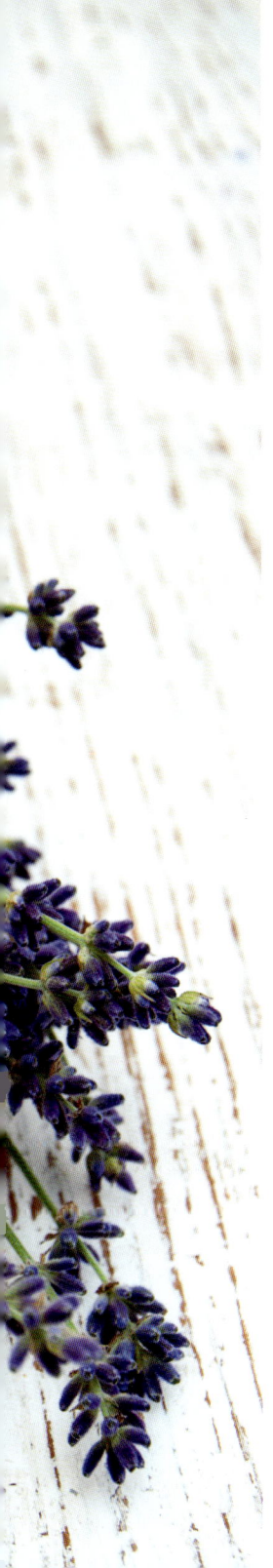

DIGESTIVE SYSTEM

Bath Salts

Ingredients:
- 3 drops Copaiba Essential Oil
- 5 drops Lavender Essential Oil
- 1/3 cup Epsom Salt
- 4 oz Glass Mason Jar

Directions:
1. Put the Epsom Salt, Copaiba and Lavender Essential Oils into a glass bowl
2. Mix the ingredients together and place the mixture into the jar
3. Add 1 tablespoon of the mixture into your bath water to support your digestive system

Drink

Ingredients:
- 1 drop Ginger Vitality Essential Oil
- 1 drop Peppermint Vitality Essential Oil
- 1 Tbsp Raw Honey
- 1 cup Water

Directions:
1. Heat up water and pour into a mug
2. Add the Essential Oils and raw honey
3. Mix together and drink to support the digestive system

Fun Easy Recipes- For Your Body Systems - 13

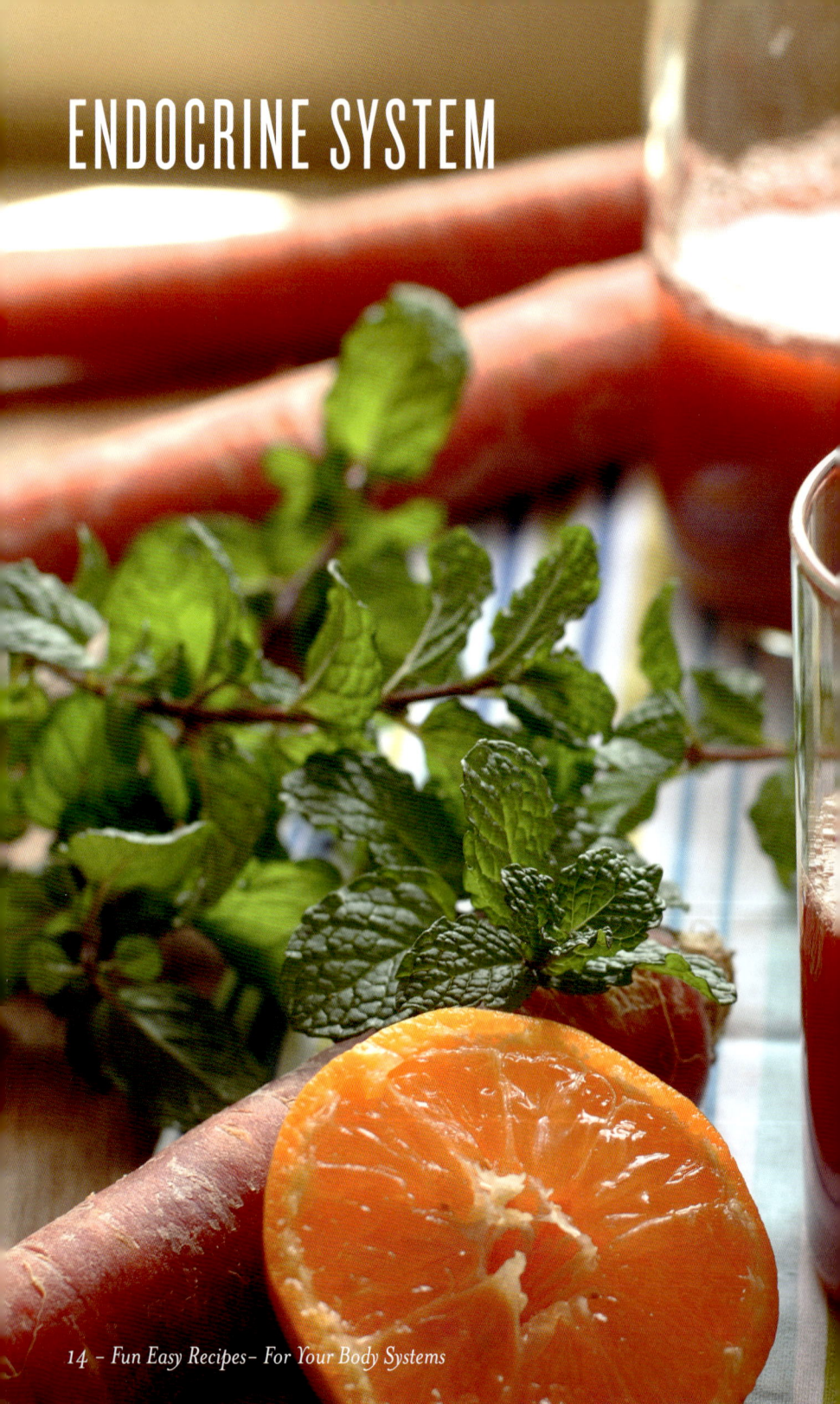
ENDOCRINE SYSTEM

14 - Fun Easy Recipes - For Your Body Systems

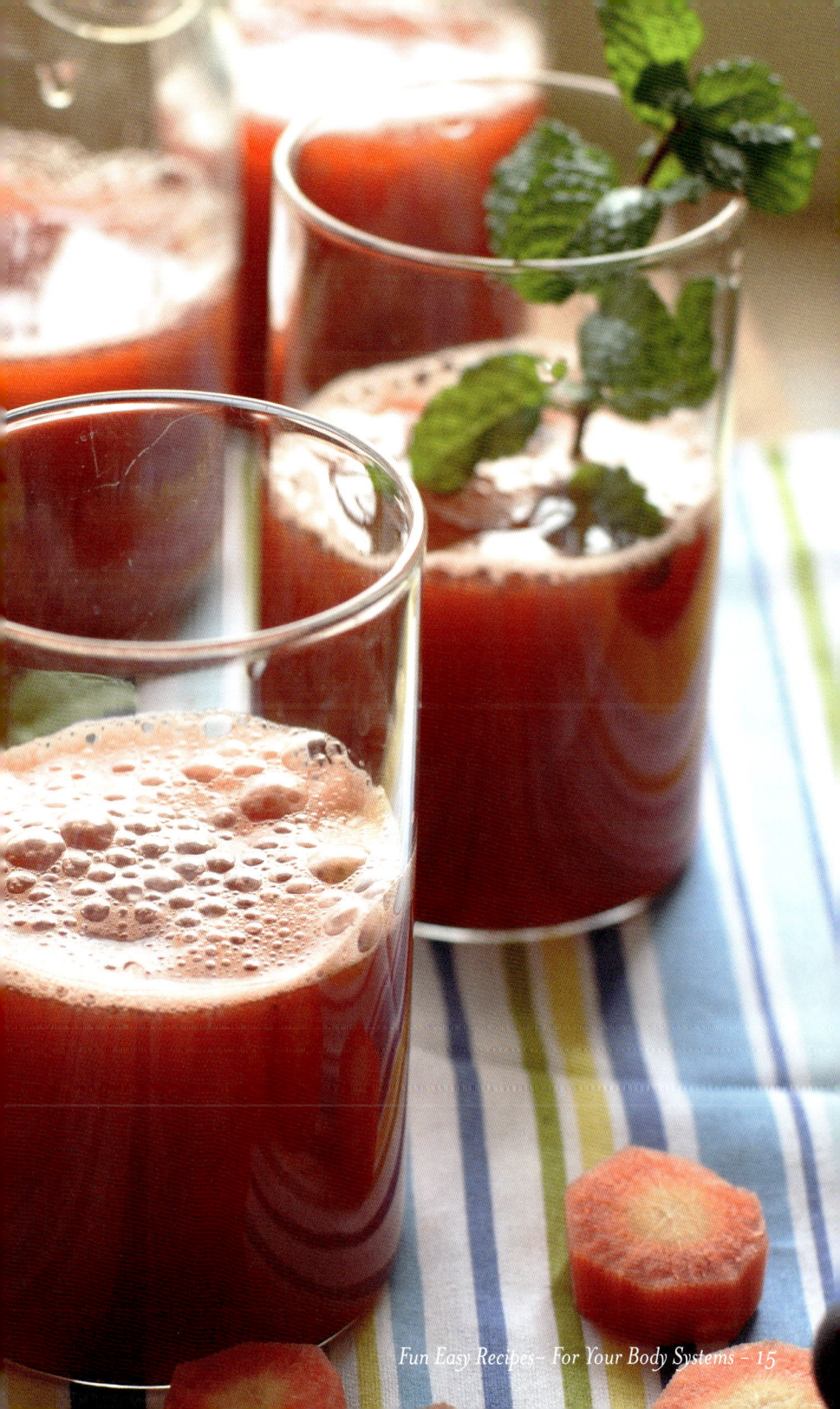

ENDOCRINE SYSTEM

Thyroid Support Roll-On

Ingredients:
- 10 drops Endoflex Essential Oil
- 5 drops Rosemary Essential Oil
- V-6 Vegetable Oil (or Liquid Coconut Oil)
- 10 mL Glass Roll-On Bottle

Directions:
1. Add the Essential Oils into the roll-on bottle
2. Fill with V-6 Vegetable Oil and put on the roll-on top
3. Apply onto your neck to support the thyroid

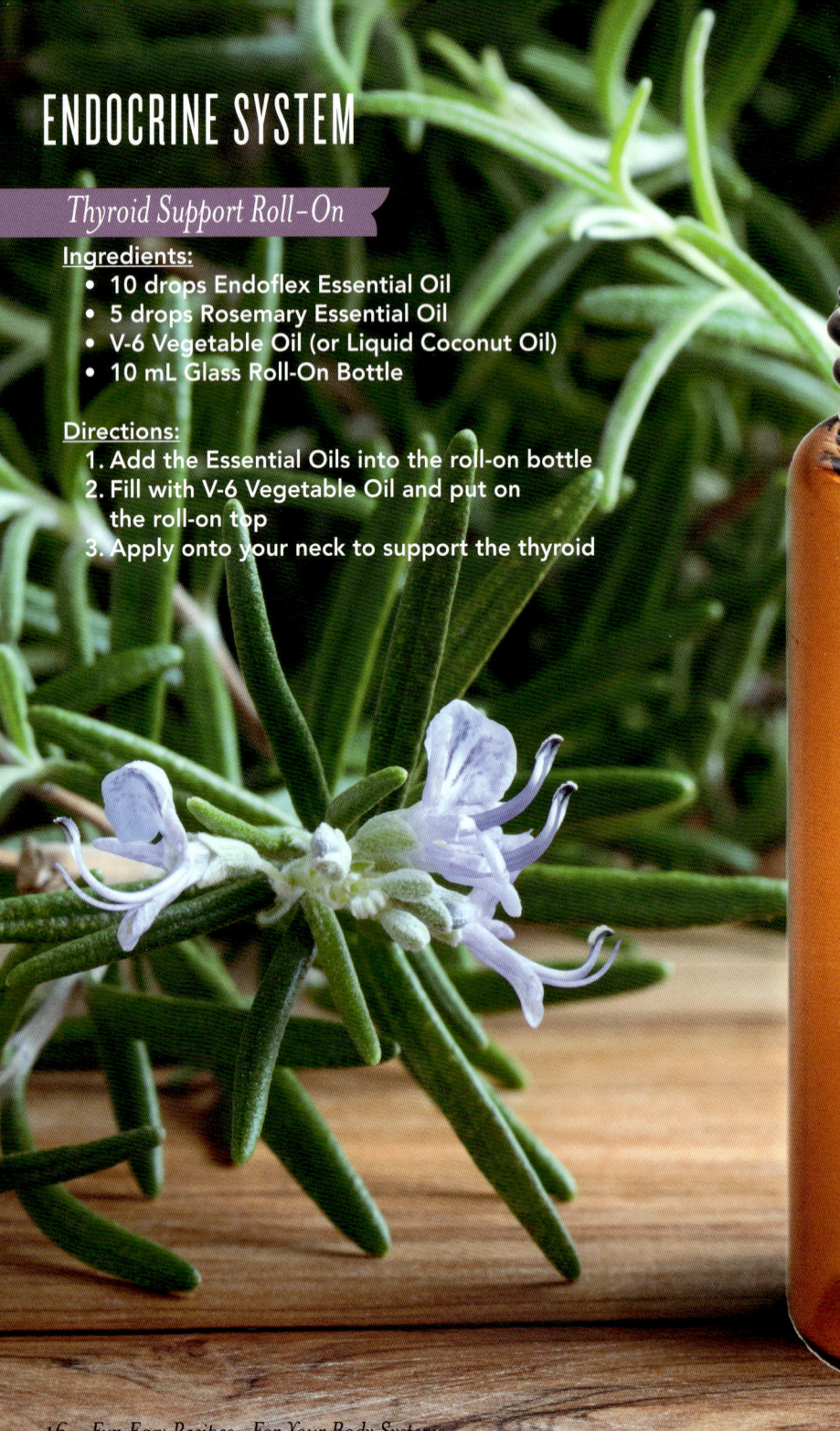

16 – Fun Easy Recipes – For Your Body Systems

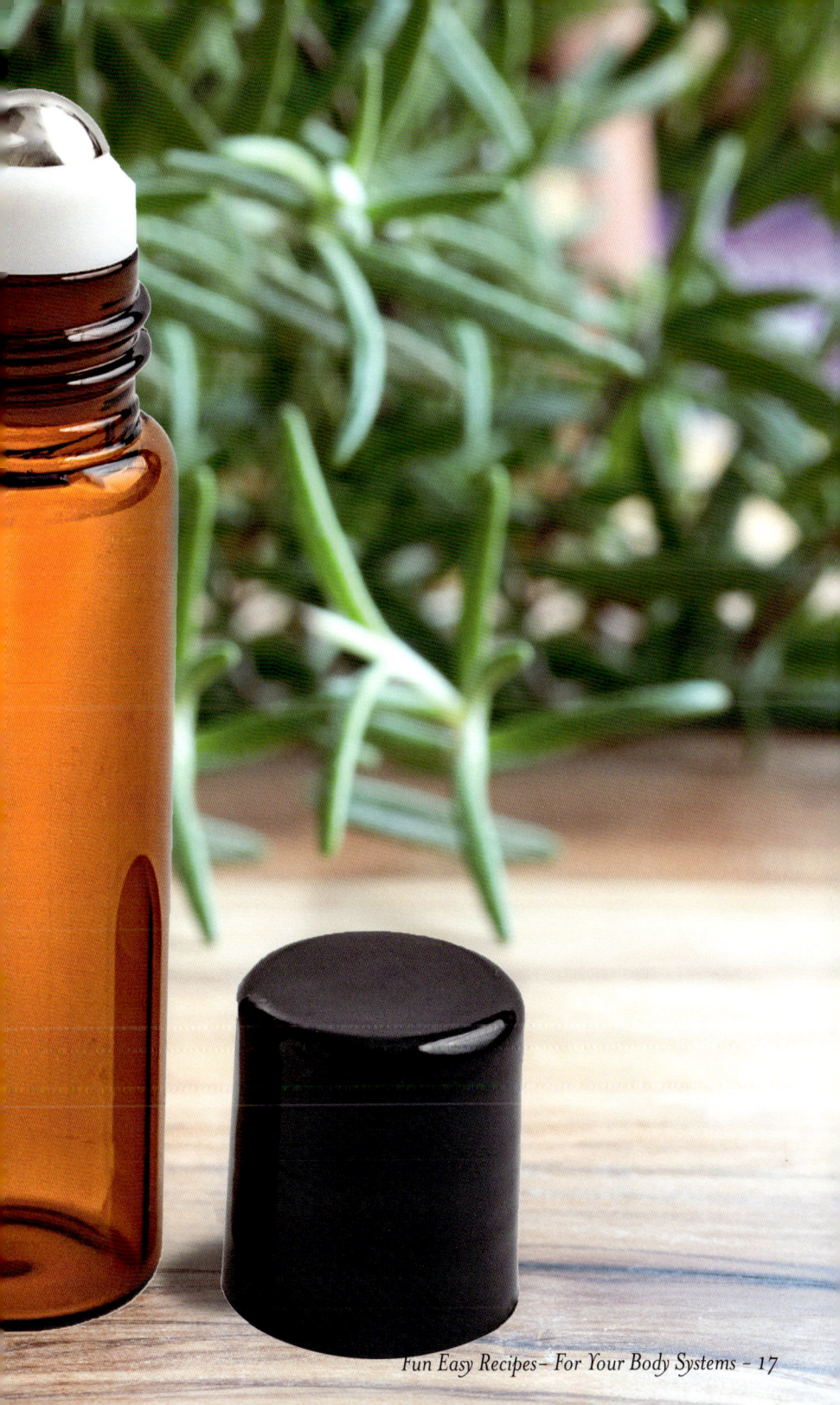

Fun Easy Recipes- For Your Body Systems - 17

ENDOCRINE SYSTEM

Capsule

Ingredients:
- 3 drops Lemon Vitality Essential Oil
- 5 drops Nutmeg Vitality Essential Oil
- Vegetable Capsule

Directions:
1. Add Lemon Vitality and Nutmeg Vitality Essential Oils into the capsule
2. Ingest one capsule to support the endocrine system as needed

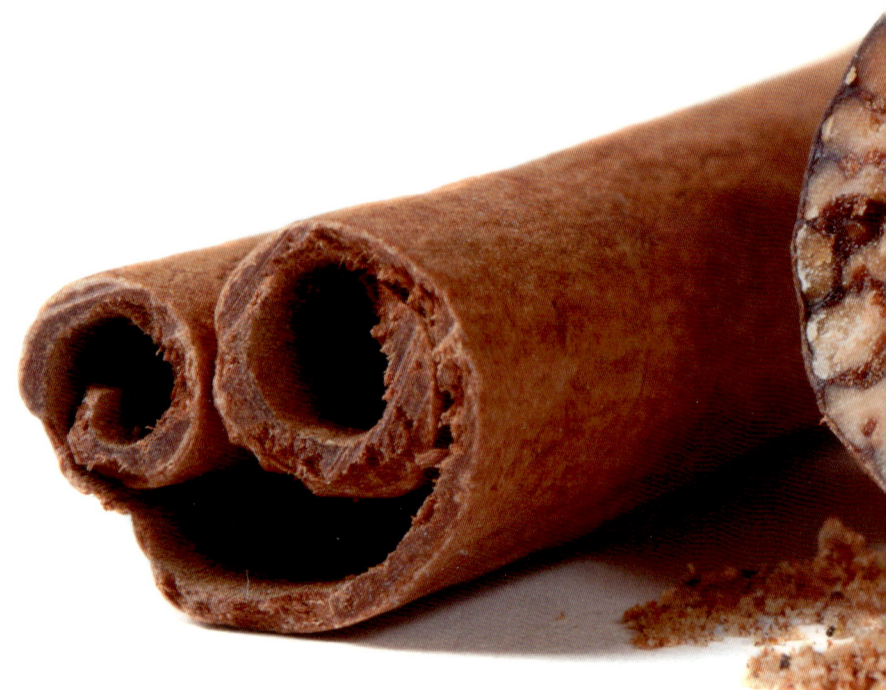

Adrenal Support Roll-On

Ingredients:
- 7 drops Nutmeg Essential Oil
- 5 drops Cinnamon Bark Essential Oil
- V-6 Vegetable Oil (or Liquid Coconut Oil)
- 10 mL Glass Roll-On Bottle

Directions:
1. Add the Essential Oils into the roll-on bottle
2. Fill with V-6 Vegetable Oil and put on the roll-on top
3. Apply onto your mid back to support the adrenal glands

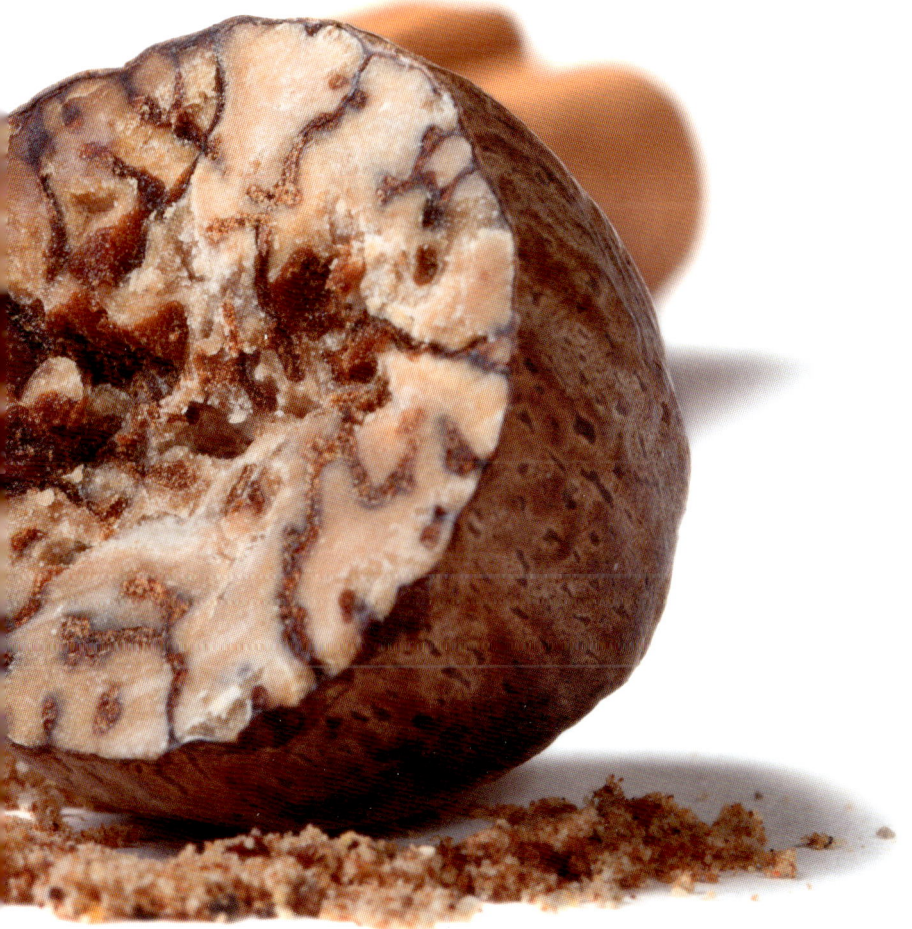

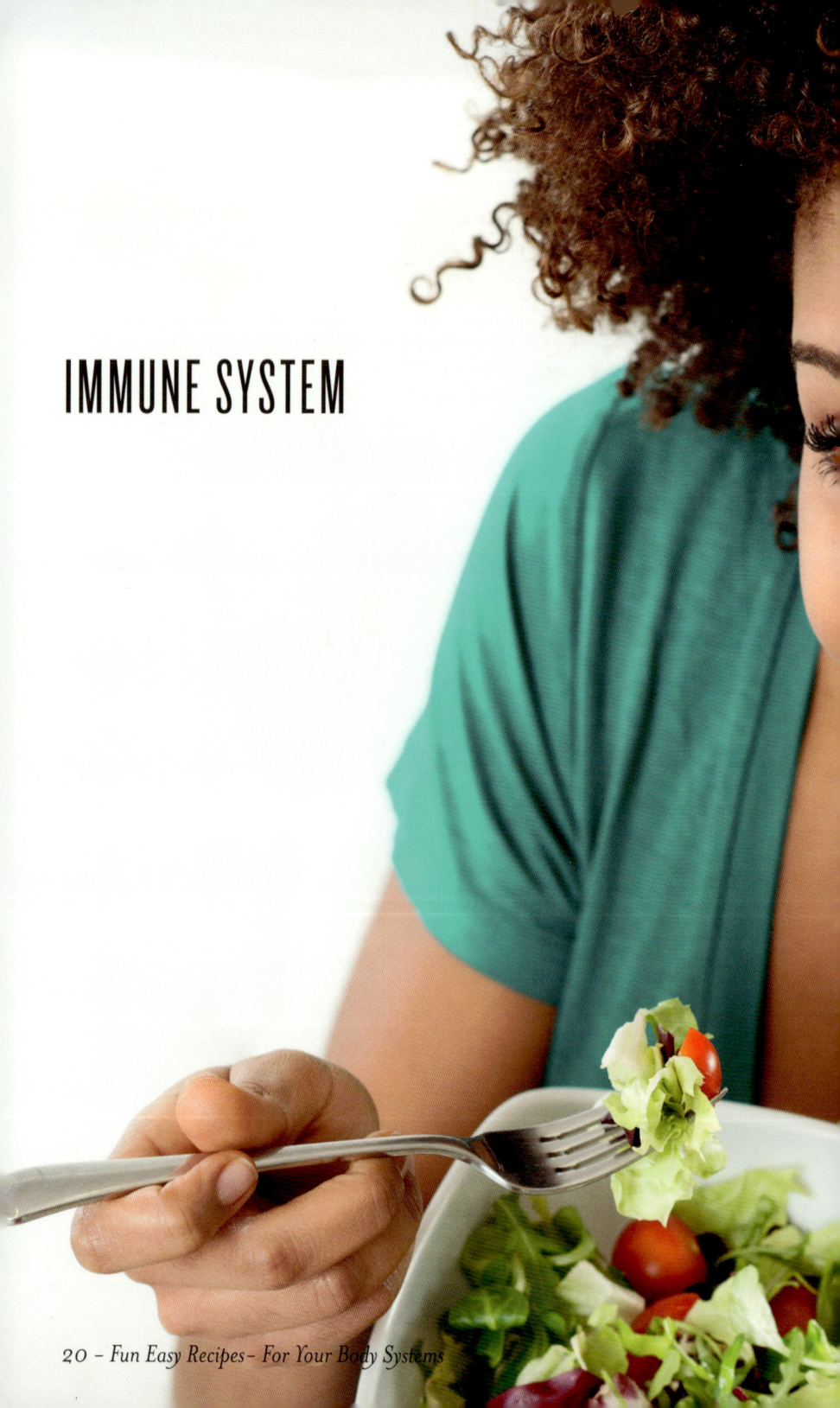

IMMUNE SYSTEM

20 - *Fun Easy Recipes- For Your Body Systems*

IMMUNE SYSTEM

Drink

Ingredients:
- 2 oz NingXia Red
- 2 drops Copaiba Vitality Essential Oil

Directions:
1. Pour NingXia Red into a shot glass
2. Add the Copaiba Vitality Essential Oil
3. Stir and drink to support the immune system

Capsule

Ingredients:
- 5 drops Thieves Vitality Essential Oil
- 5 drops Lemon Vitality Essential Oil
- Vegetable Capsule

Directions:
1. Add Thieves Vitality and Lemon Vitality Essential Oils into the capsule
2. Ingest one capsule for immune support as needed

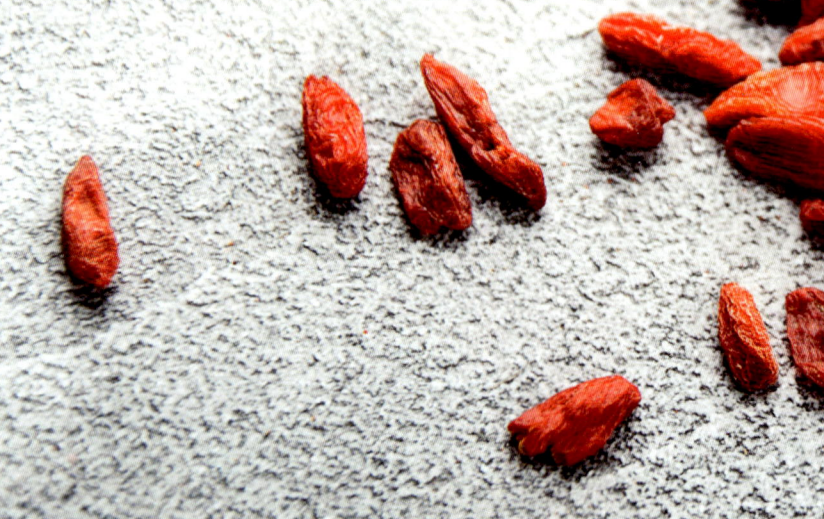

22 – *Fun Easy Recipes– For Your Body Systems*

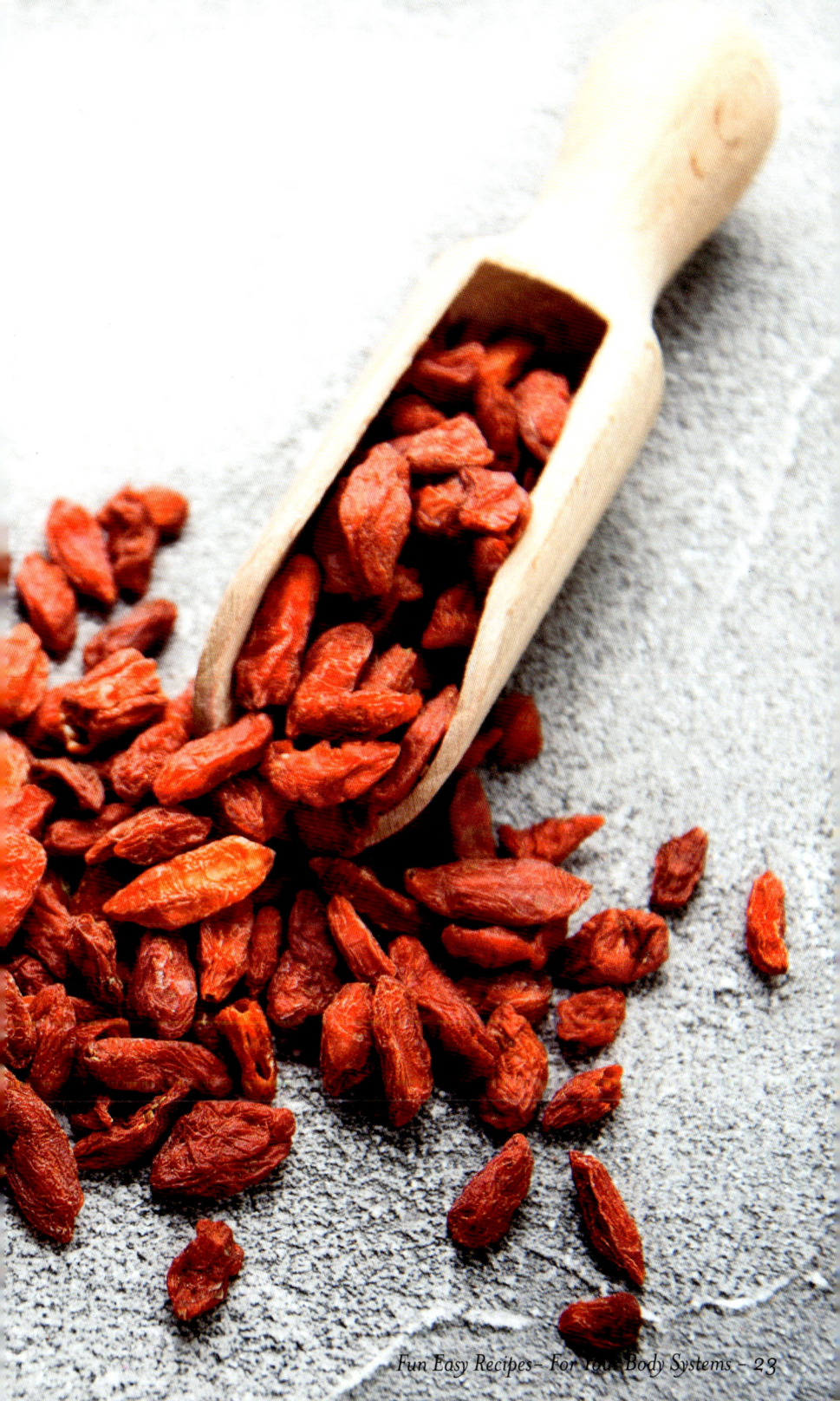

IMMUNE SYSTEM

Diffuser Blend

Ingredients:
- 3 drops Thieves Essential Oil
- 2 drops Raven Essential Oil
- Water
- Diffuser

Directions:
1. Add water to the fill line of the diffuser
2. Put Thieves and Raven Essential Oils into the water
3. Put the top of the diffuser on and press the on button
4. Enjoy the refreshing scent while supporting the immune system

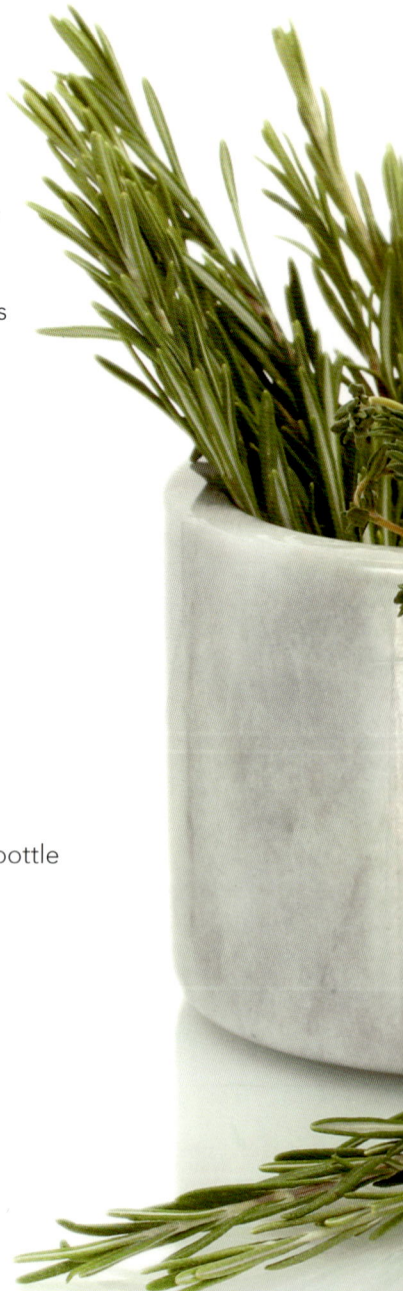

Roll-On

Ingredients:
- 8 drops Thieves Essential Oil
- 8 drops ImmuPower Essential Oil
- V-6 Vegetable Oil (or Liquid Coconut Oil)
- 10 mL Glass Roll-On Bottle

Directions:
1. Add the Essential Oils into the roll-on bottle
2. Fill with V-6 Vegetable Oil and put on the roll-on top
3. Apply onto your spine or feet daily to support the immune system

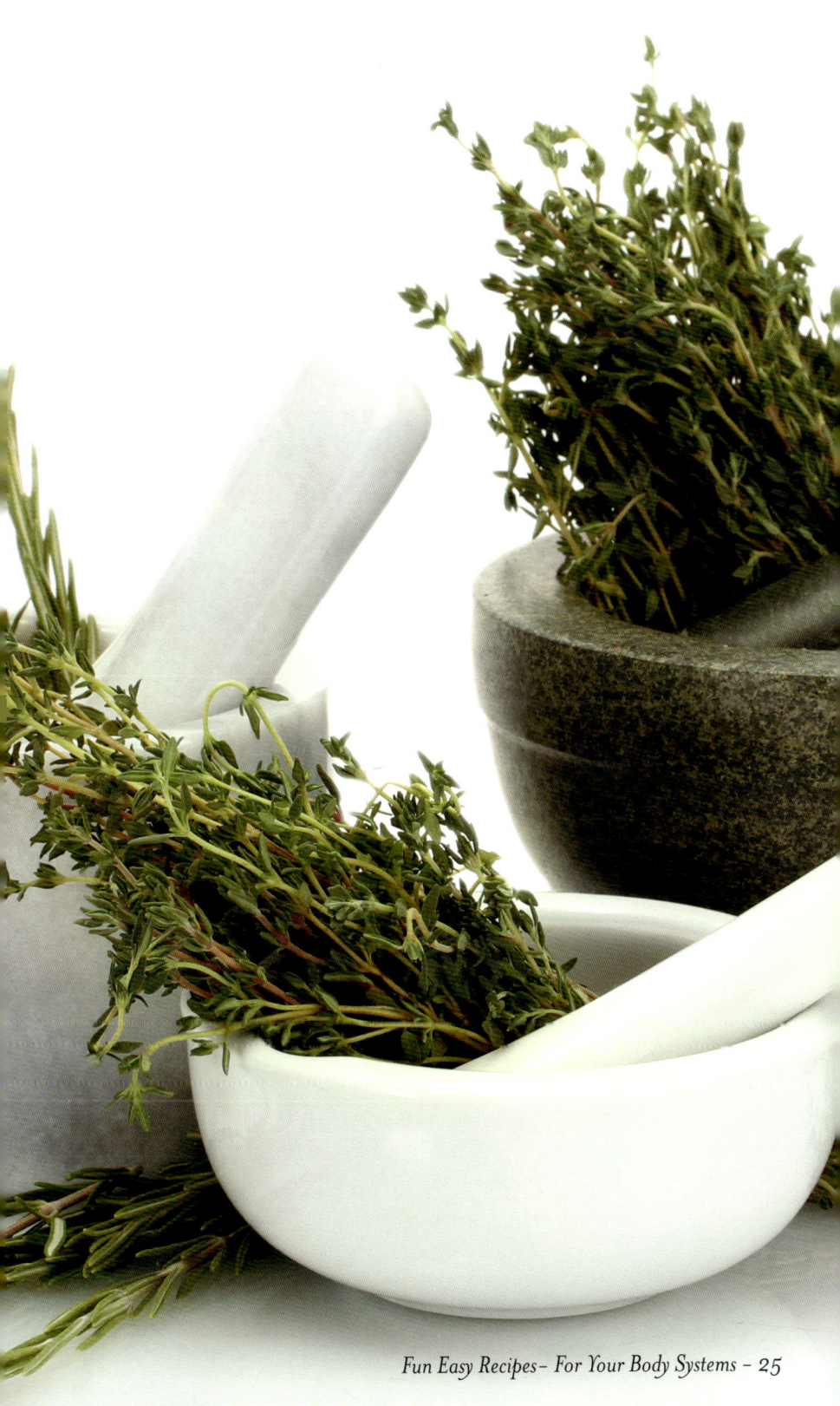
Fun Easy Recipes- For Your Body Systems - 25

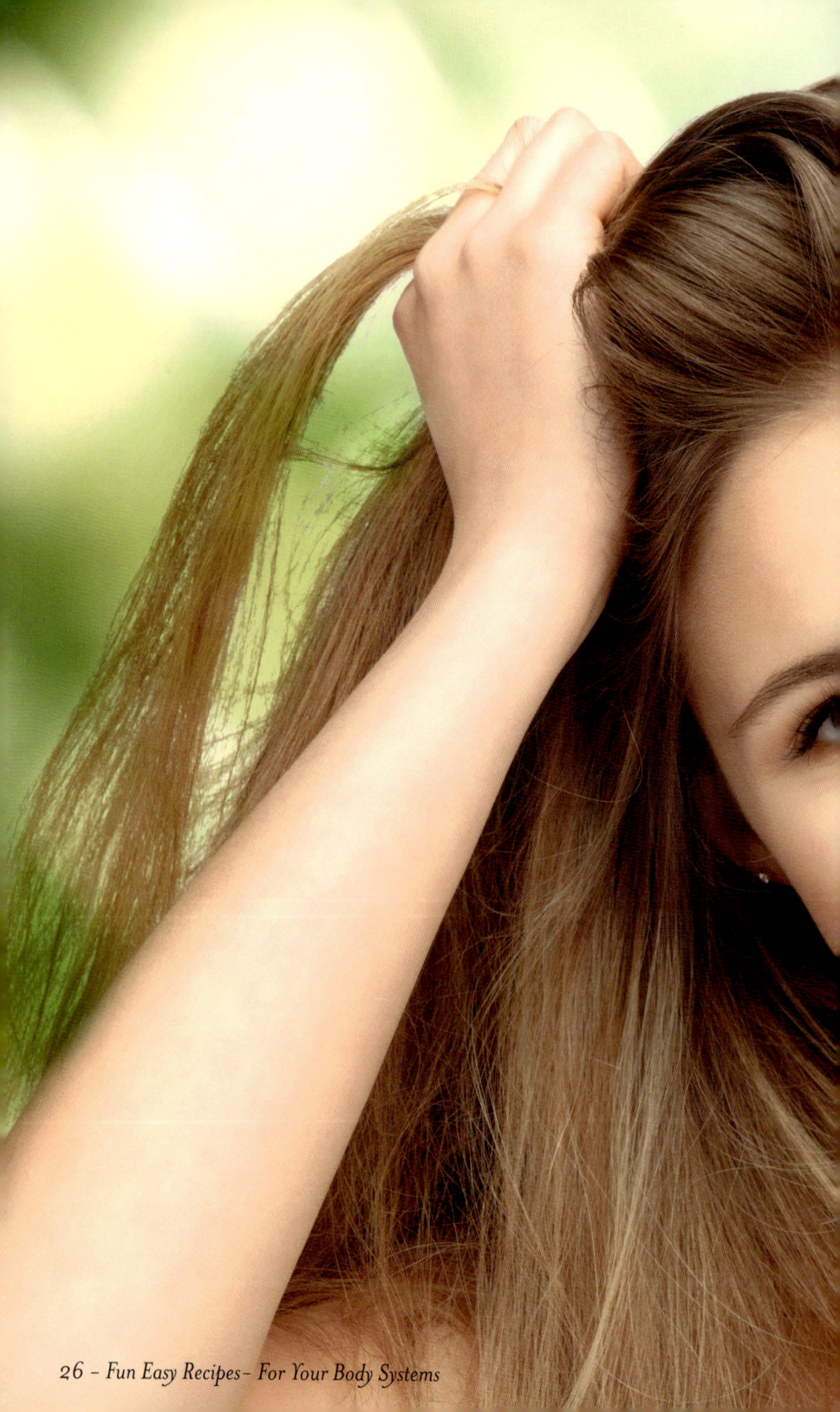

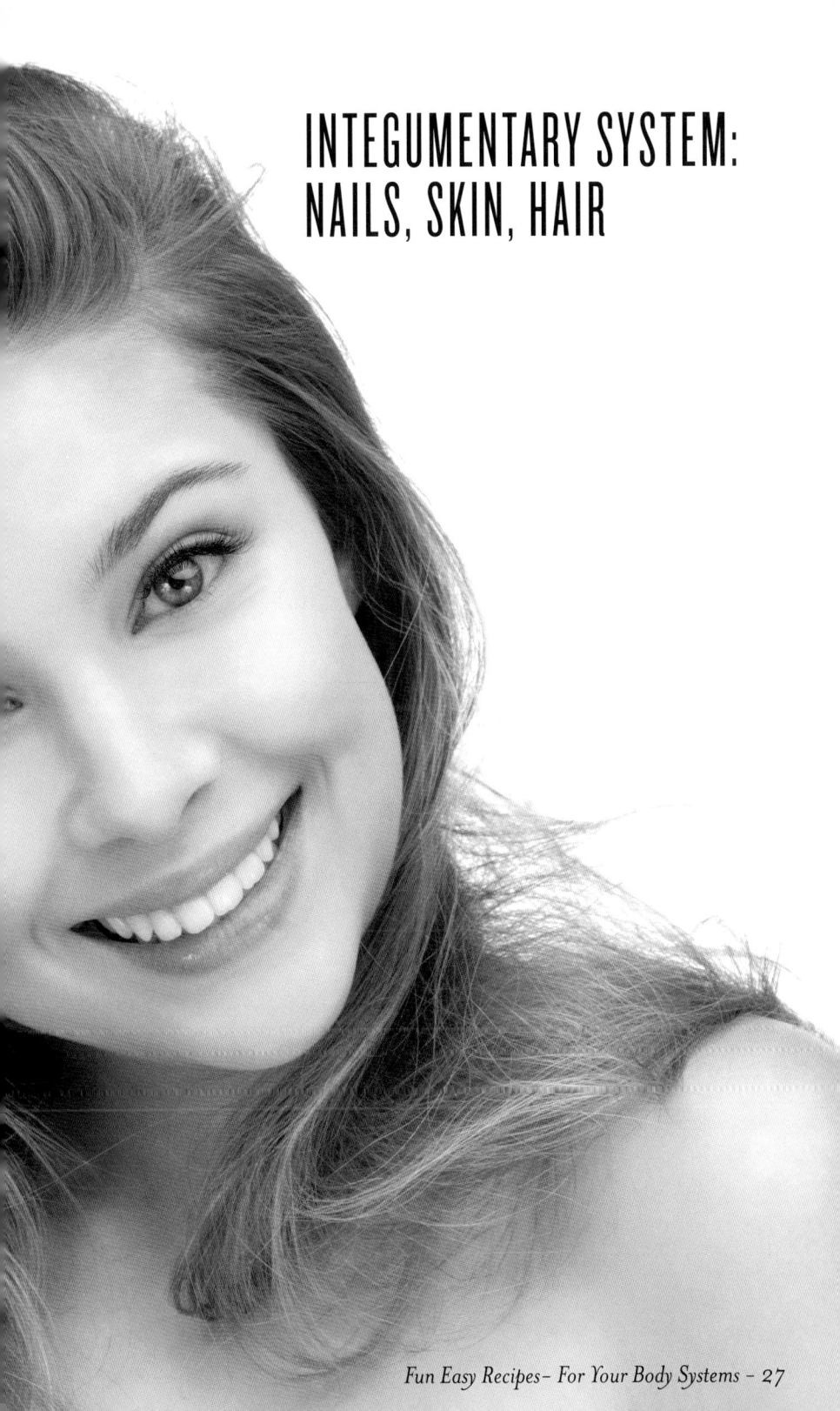

INTEGUMENTARY SYSTEM: NAILS, SKIN, HAIR

INTEGUMENTARY SYSTEM

Nail Strengthening Roll-On

Ingredients:
- 10 drops Lavender Essential Oil
- 10 drops Myrrh Essential Oil
- 10 drops Frankincense Essential Oil
- V-6 Vegetable Oil (or Liquid Coconut Oil)
- 10 mL Glass Roll-On Bottle

Directions:
1. Add the Essential Oils into the roll-on bottle
2. Fill with V-6 Vegetable Oil and put on the roll-on top
3. Apply onto your nails in the morning and at night to strengthen them

Sugar Scrub - Skin Support

Ingredients:
- 4 drops Frankincense Essential Oil
- 4 drops Tea Tree Essential Oil
- 1/2 cup Raw Sugar
- 1/4 cup Virgin Coconut Oil
- 4 oz Glass Mason Jar

Directions:
1. Put the Raw Sugar, Coconut Oil and Essential Oils into a glass bowl
2. Mix the ingredients together
3. Place the mixture into the jar
4. Use this scrub to exfoliate your hands or body

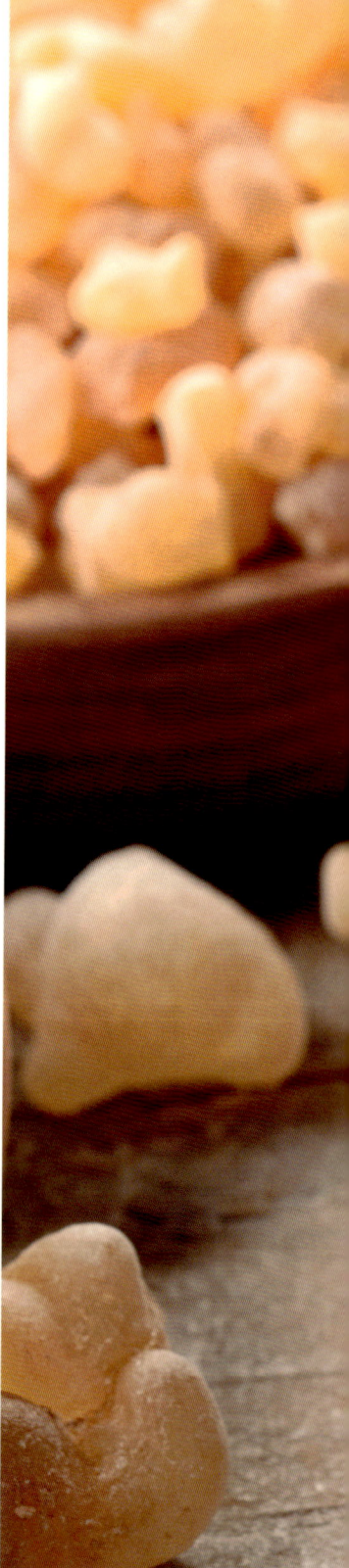

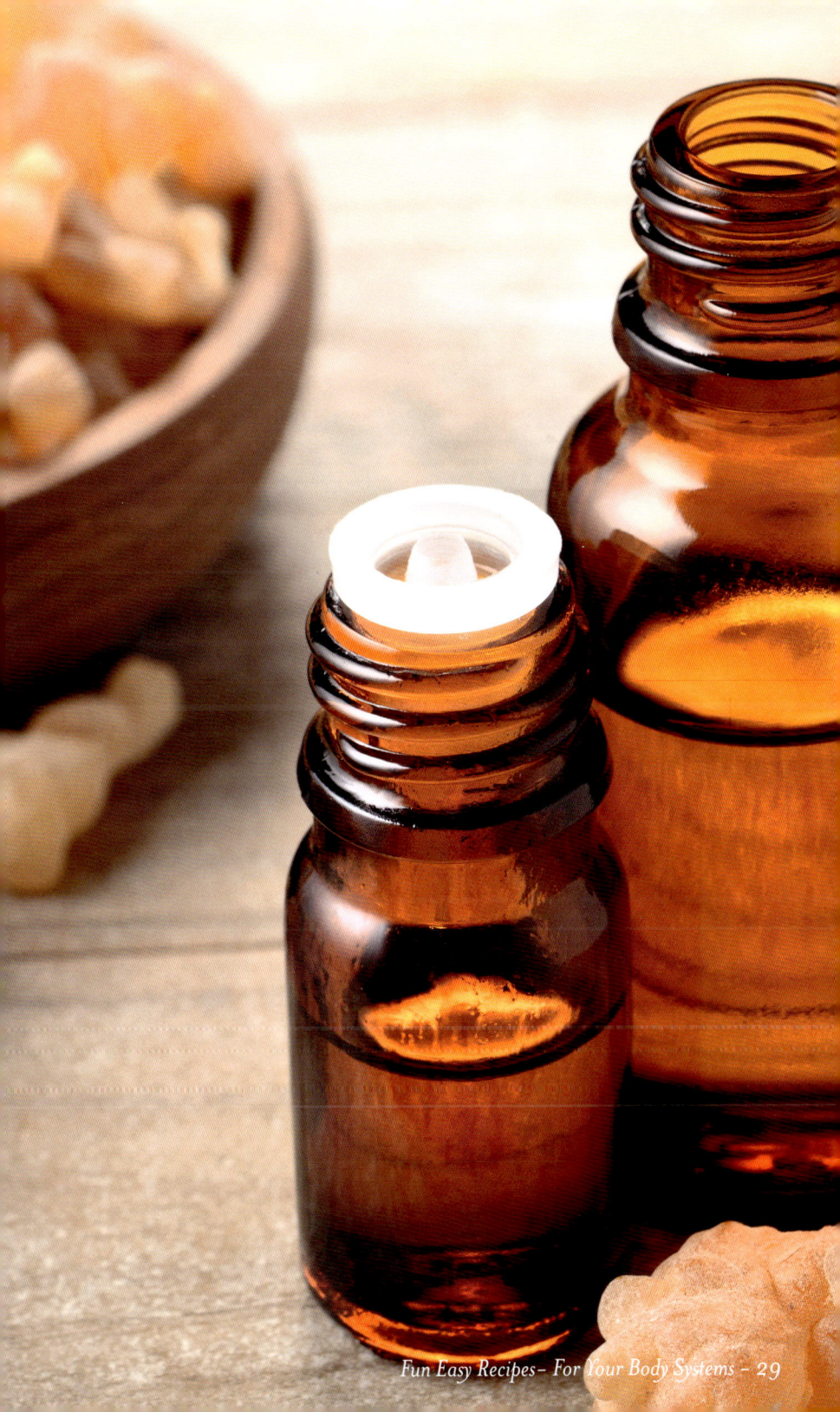

INTEGUMENTARY SYSTEM

After Shave Ointment

Ingredients:
- 4 drops Lavender Essential Oil
- 3 drops Melrose Essential Oil
- 1/3 cup Virgin Coconut Oil
- 1 Tbsp Aloe Vera
- 4 oz Glass Mason Jar

Directions:
1. Put the Coconut Oil, Aloe Vera, Lavender and Melrose Essential Oils into a glass bowl
2. Mix the ingredients together and place the mixture into the jar
3. Apply a small amount of mixture onto your skin after shaving

Hair Strengthening Spray

Ingredients:
- 6 drops Rosemary Essential Oil
- 6 drops Lavender Essential Oil
- 6 drops Cedarwood Essential Oil
- Water
- 2 oz Glass Spray Bottle

Directions:
1. Add the Essential Oils into the spray bottle
2. Fill with water and put on the spray bottle top
3. Shake well before spraying onto your hair at night. Wash your hair in the morning.

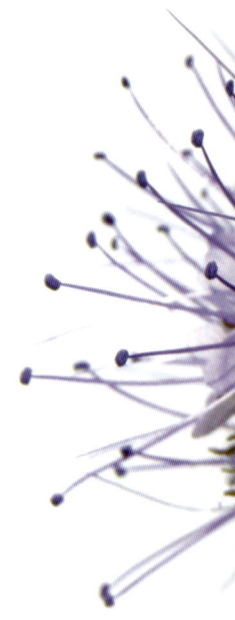

Nourishing Hair Balm

Ingredients:
- 4 drops Lavender Essential Oil
- 4 drops Cedarwood Essential Oil
- 3 drops Geranium Essential Oil
- 1/3 cup Virgin Coconut Oil
- 4 oz Glass Mason Jar

Directions:
1. Add Lavender, Cedarwood, and Geranium Essential Oils and Coconut Oil into a glass bowl
2. Mix the ingredients together
3. Place the mixture into the jar. Apply a small amount of the mixture to your hair at night. Wash your hair in the morning.

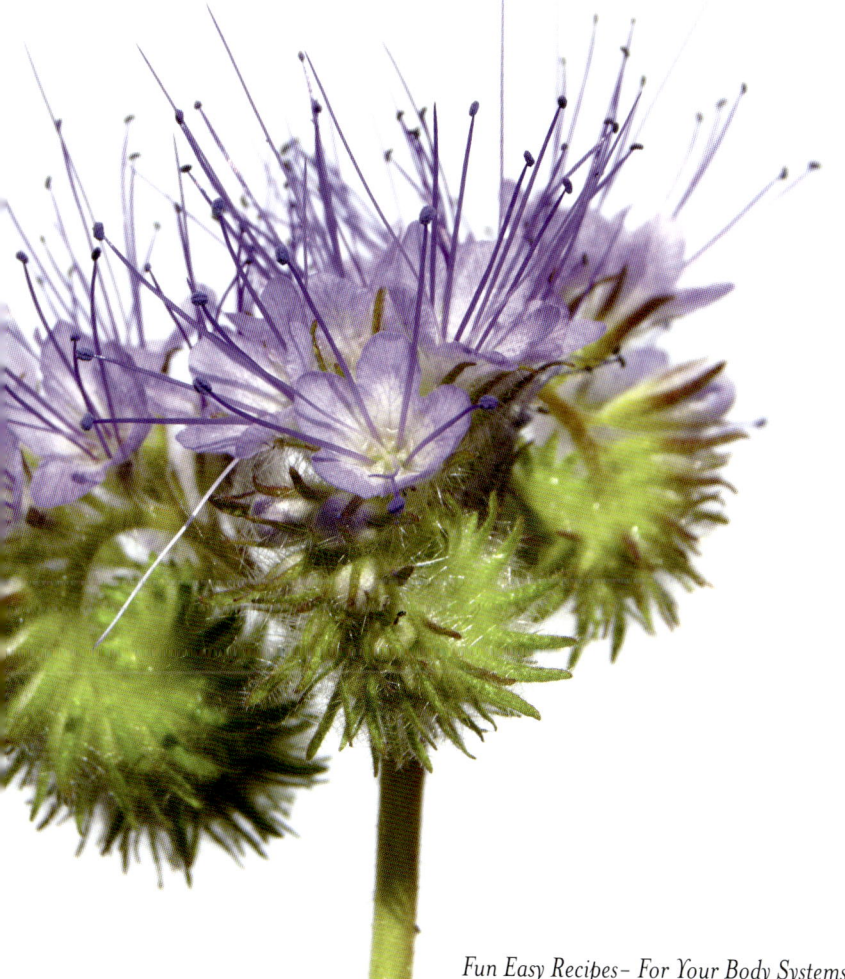

Fun Easy Recipes- For Your Body Systems

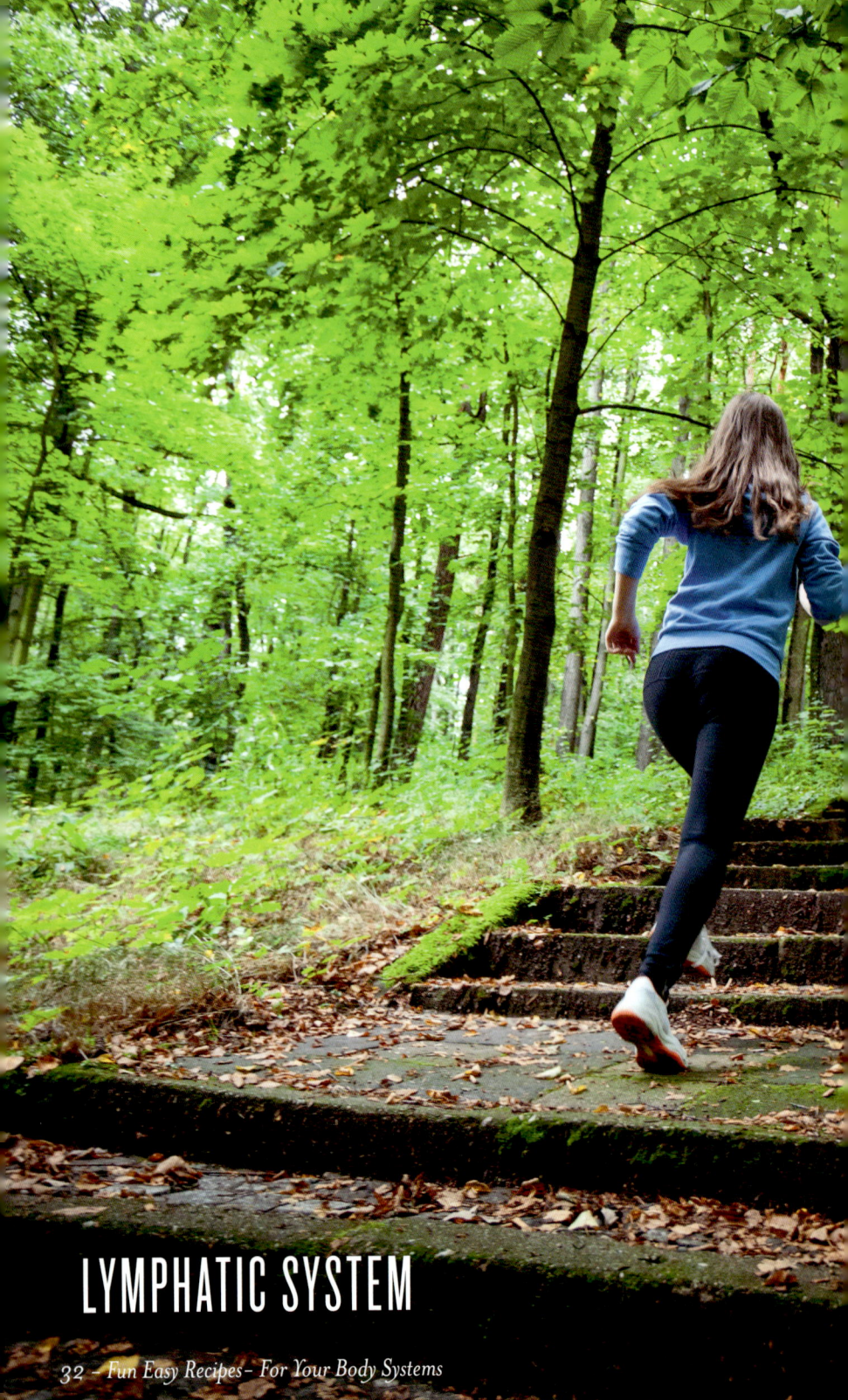

LYMPHATIC SYSTEM

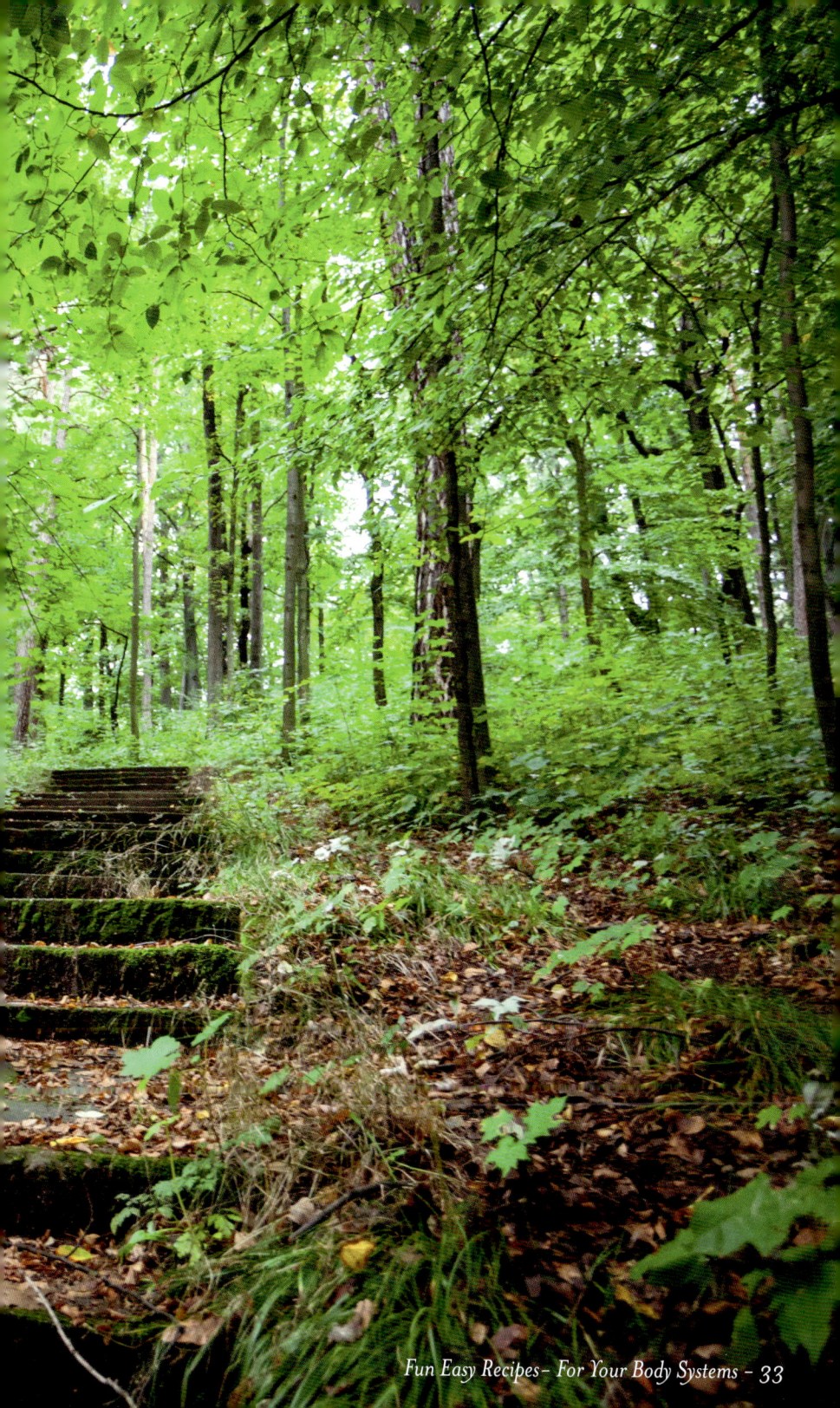

LYMPHATIC SYSTEM

Roll-On

Ingredients:
- 6 drops Cypress Essential Oil
- 6 drops Lemongrass Essential Oil
- V-6 Vegetable Oil (or Liquid Coconut Oil)
- 10 mL Glass Roll-On Bottle

Directions:
1. Add the Essential Oils into the roll-on bottle
2. Fill with V-6 Vegetable Oil and put on the roll-on top
3. Apply onto the area of need to support circulation

Bath Salts

Ingredients:
- 4 drops Ledum Essential Oil
- 4 drops JuvaFlex Essential Oil
- 1/3 cup Epsom Salt
- 4 oz Glass Mason Jar

Directions:
1. Put the Epsom Salt, Ledum and JuvaFlex Essential Oils into a glass bowl
2. Mix the ingredients together and place the mixture into the jar
3. Add 1 tablespoon of the mixture into your bath water to support the lymphatic system

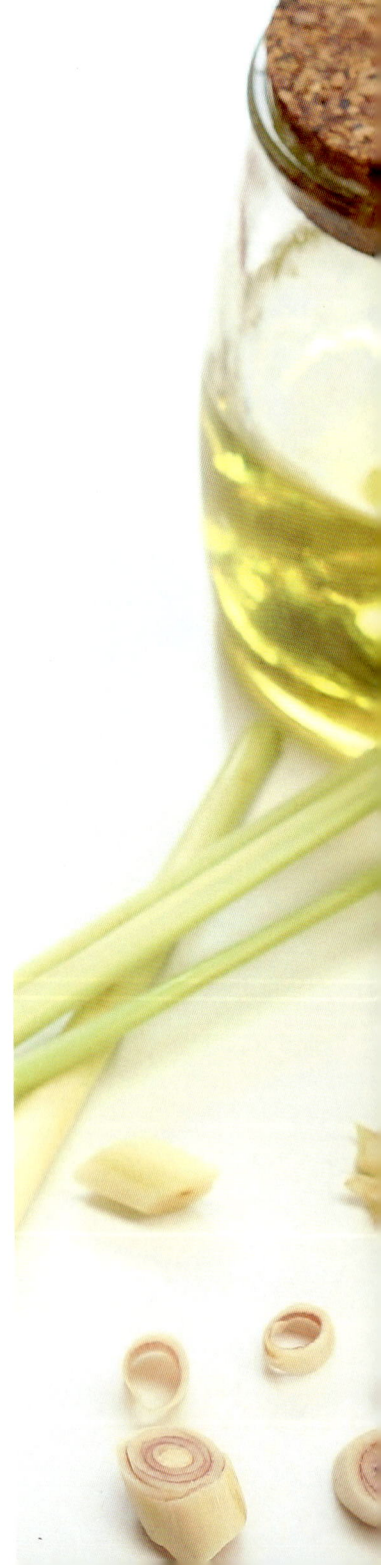

Fun Easy Recipes- For Your Body Systems - 35

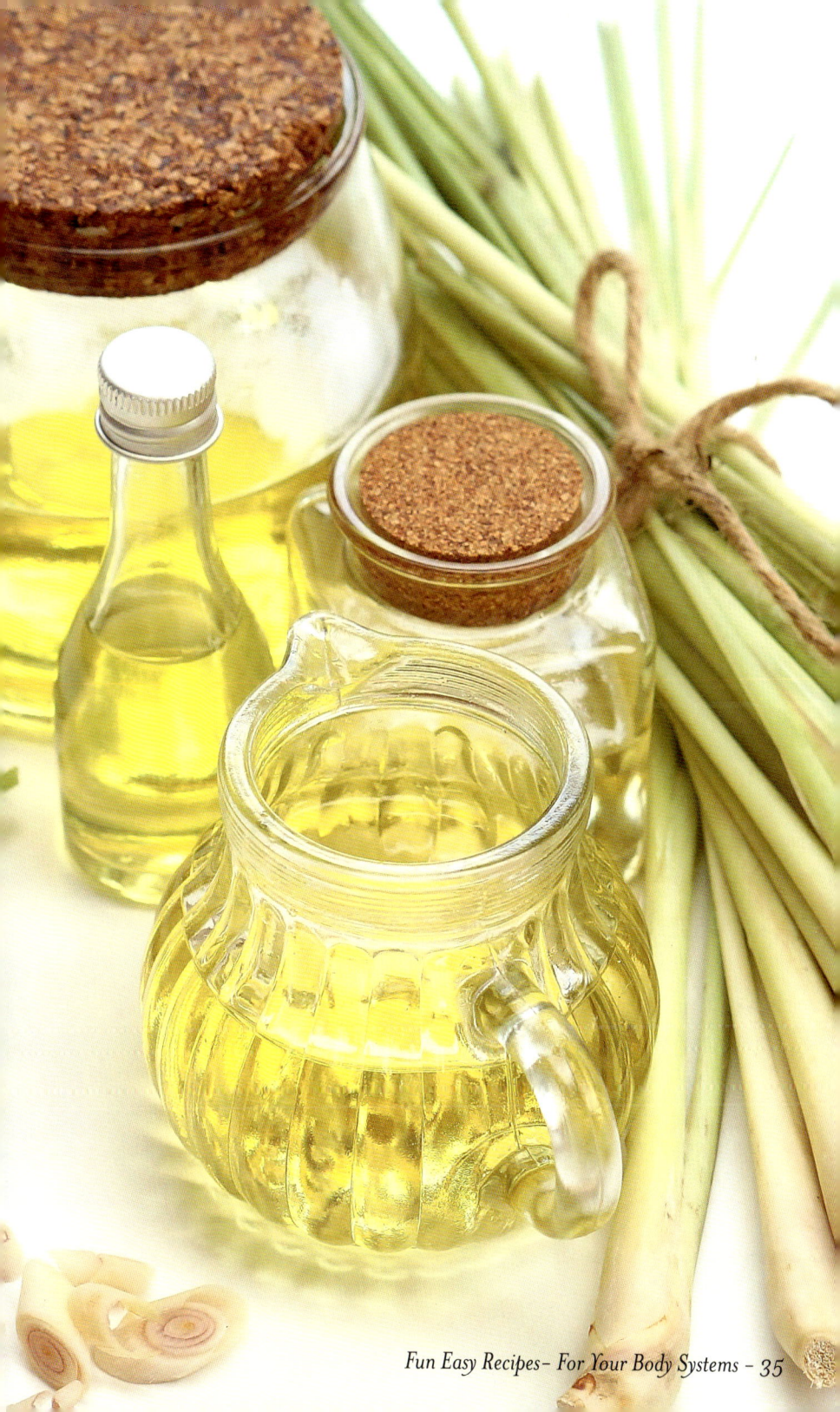

LYMPHATIC SYSTEM

Body Rub

Ingredients:
- 6 drops Cypress Essential Oil
- 4 drops Ledum Essential Oil
- 4 drops Lemon Essential Oil
- 1/3 cup Virgin Coconut Oil
- 4 oz Glass Mason Jar

Directions:
1. Add the Coconut Oil, Cypress, Ledum, and Lemon Essential Oils into a glass bowl
2. Mix the ingredients together
3. Place the mixture into the jar and apply to the area needing circulatory support

Fun Easy Recipes- For Your Body Systems - 37

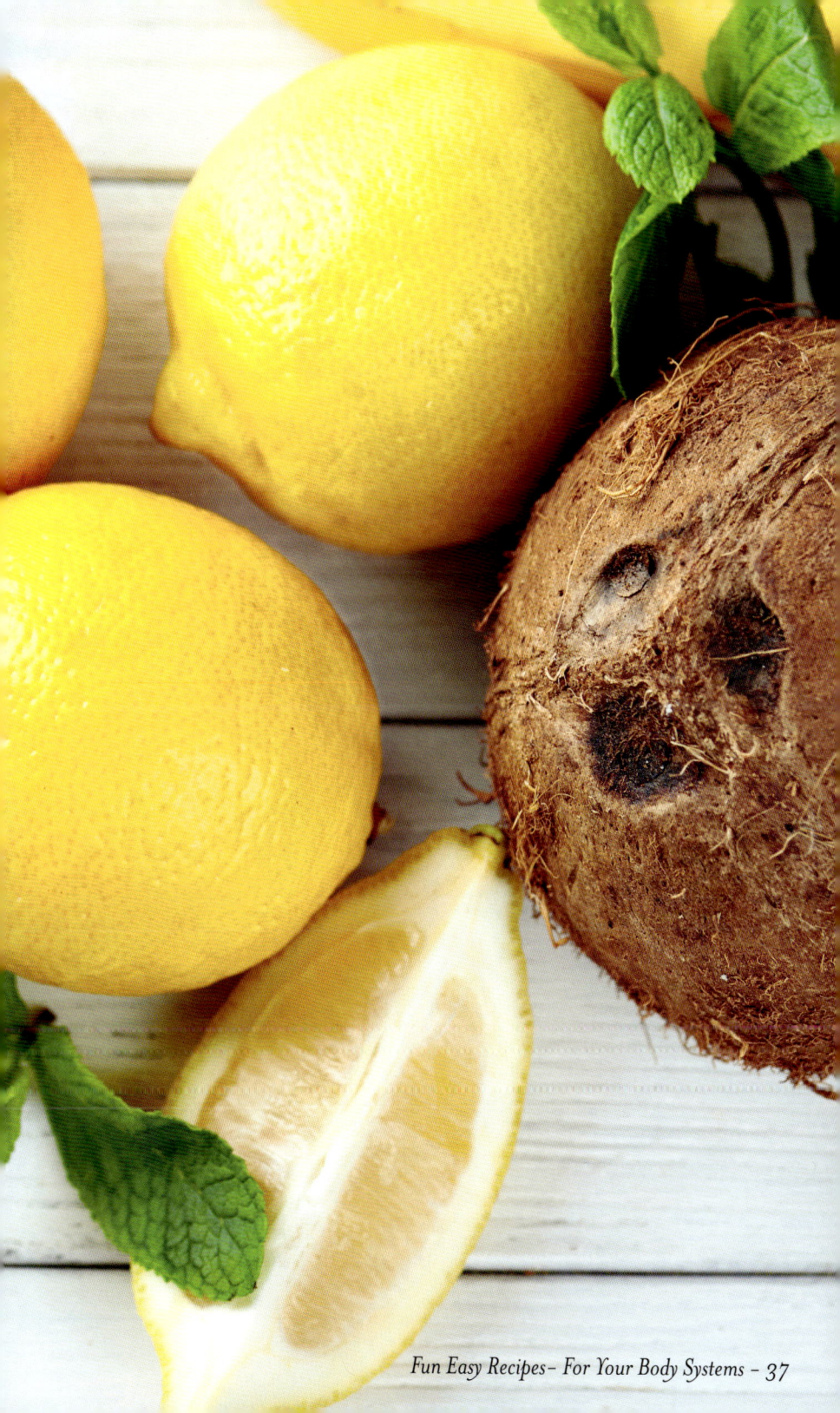

38 - Fun Easy Recipes - For Your Body Systems

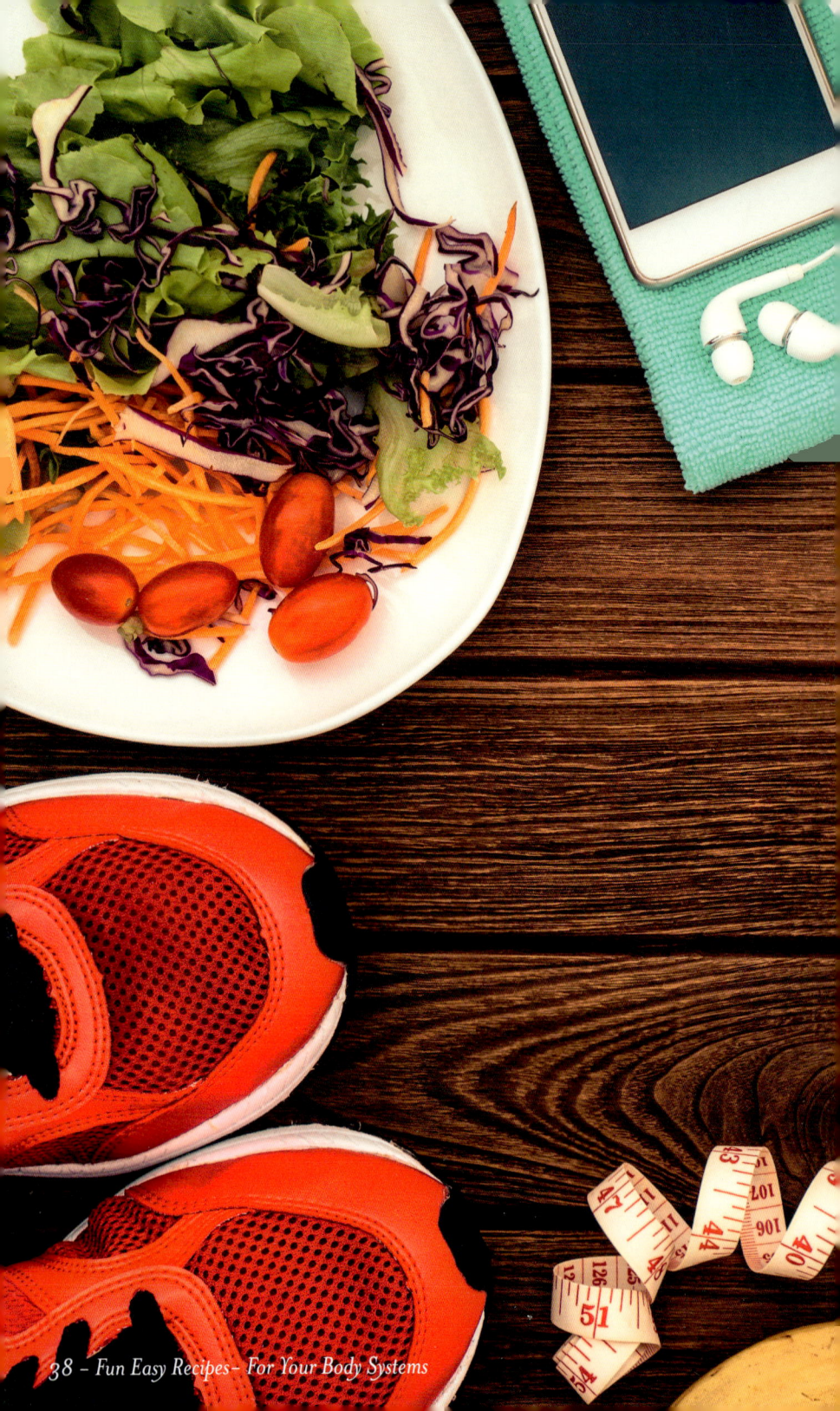

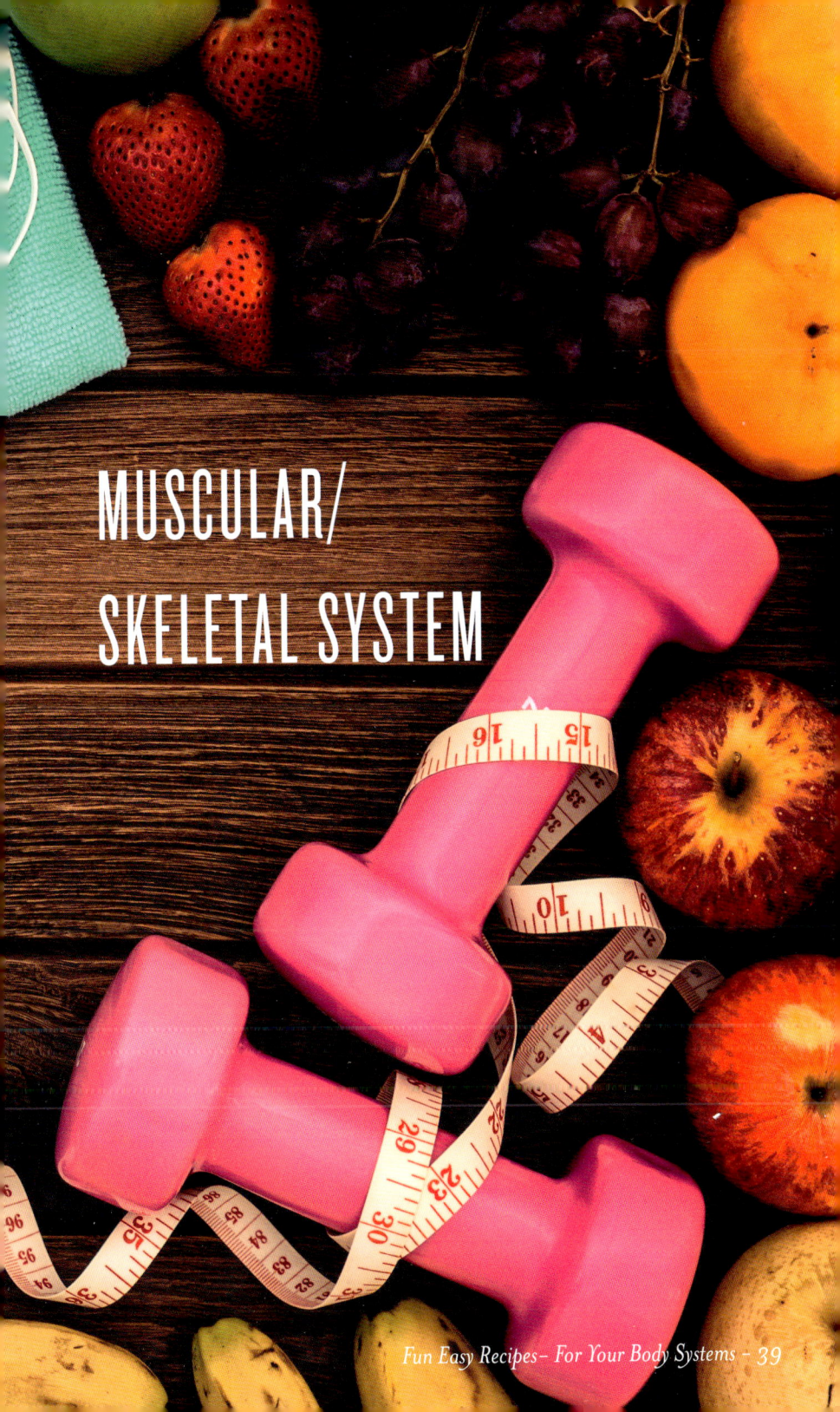

MUSCULAR/ SKELETAL SYSTEM

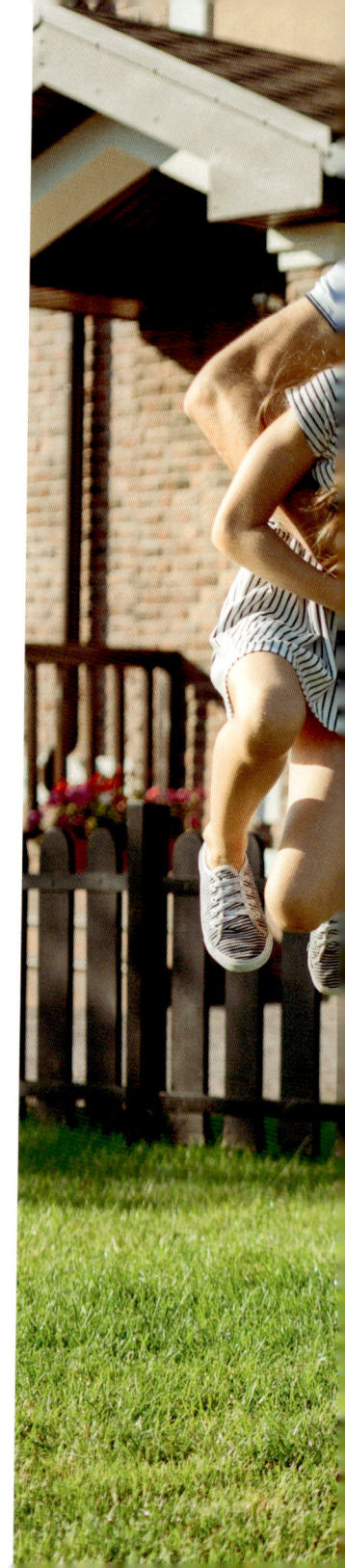

MUSCULAR/SKELETAL SYSTEM

Capsule

Ingredients:
- 6 drops Copaiba Vitality Essential Oil
- 4 drops Frankincense Vitality Essential Oil
- Vegetable Capsule

Directions:
1. Add the Essential Oils into the capsule
2. Ingest one capsule for muscle and joint support as needed

Roll-On

Ingredients:
- 7 drops Valor Essential Oil
- 7 drops PanAway Essential Oil
- V-6 Vegetable Oil (or Liquid Coconut Oil)
- 10 mL Glass Roll-On Bottle

Directions:
1. Add Valor and PanAway Essential Oils into the roll-on bottle
2. Fill with V-6 Vegetable Oil and put on the roll-on top
3. Apply onto your body where you need muscular/skeletal support

Fun Easy Recipes- For Your Body Systems – 41

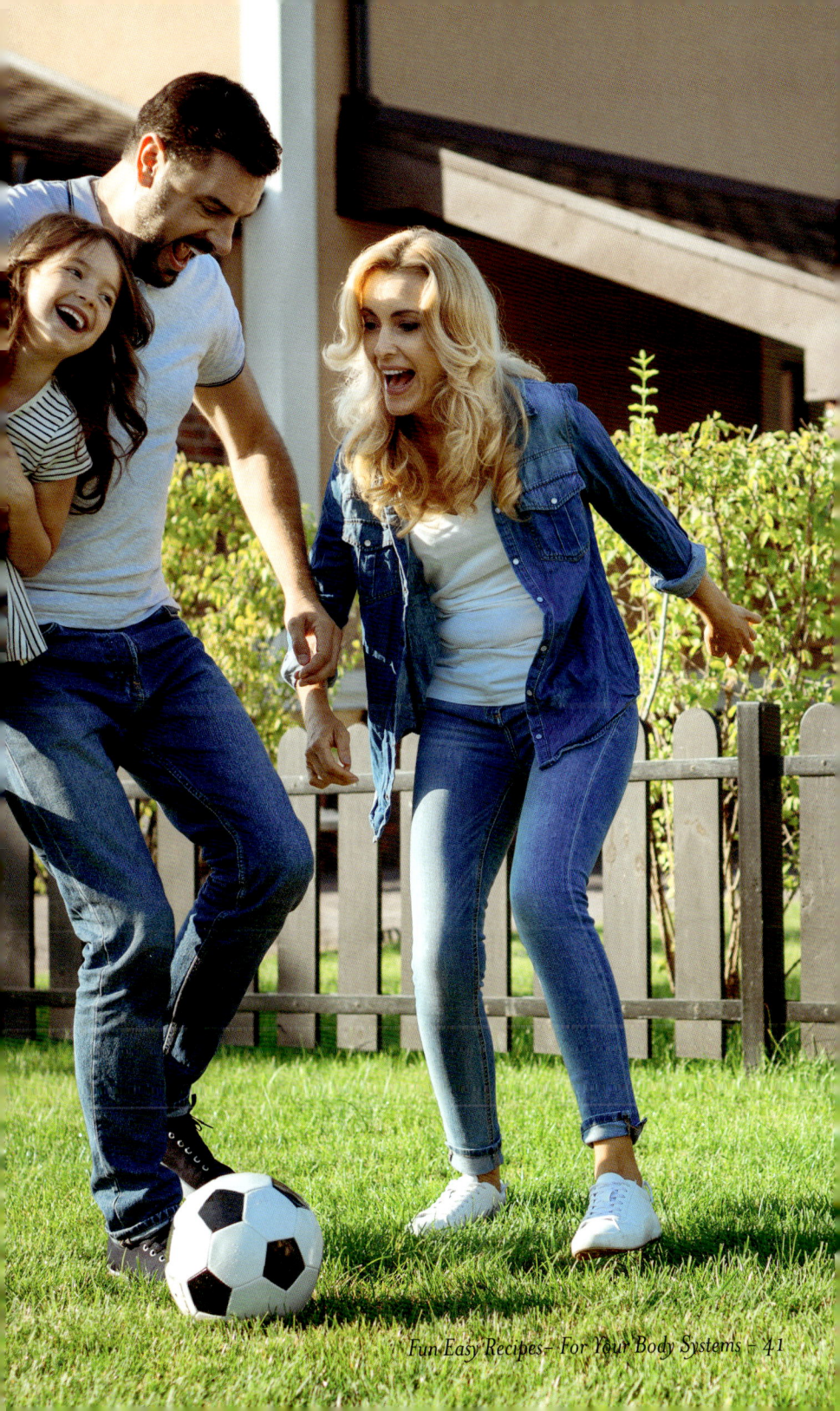

MUSCULAR/SKELETAL SYSTEM

Body Rub

Ingredients:
- 4 drops Wintergreen Essential Oil
- 4 drops Marjoram Essential Oil
- 4 drops Copaiba Essential Oil
- 1/3 cup Virgin Coconut Oil
- 4 oz Glass Mason Jar

Directions:
1. Add the Coconut Oil, Wintergreen, Marjoram, and Copaiba Essential Oils into a glass bowl
2. Mix the ingredients together
3. Place the mixture into the jar.
   Apply onto your muscles as needed.

Fun Easy Recipes- For Your Body Systems - 43

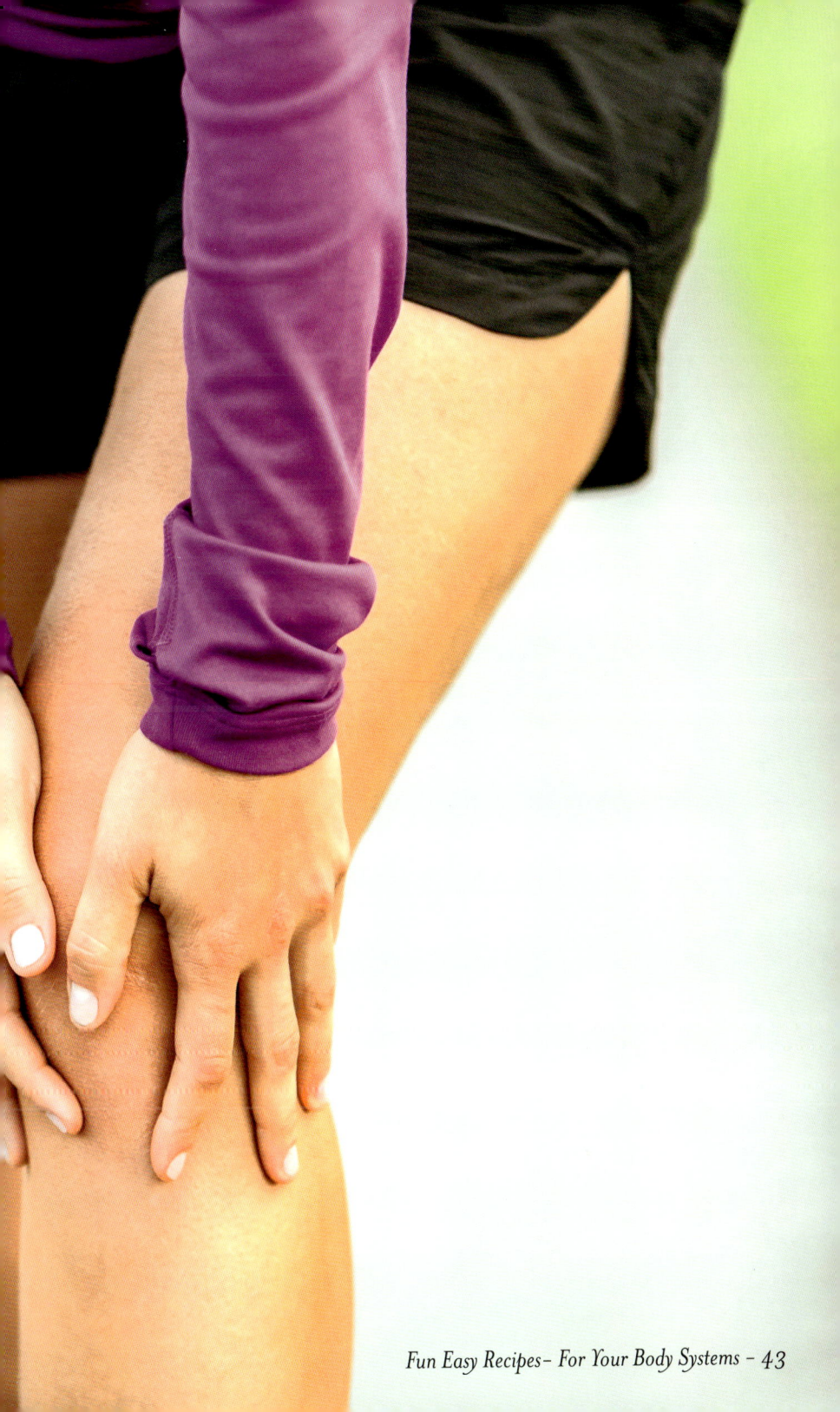

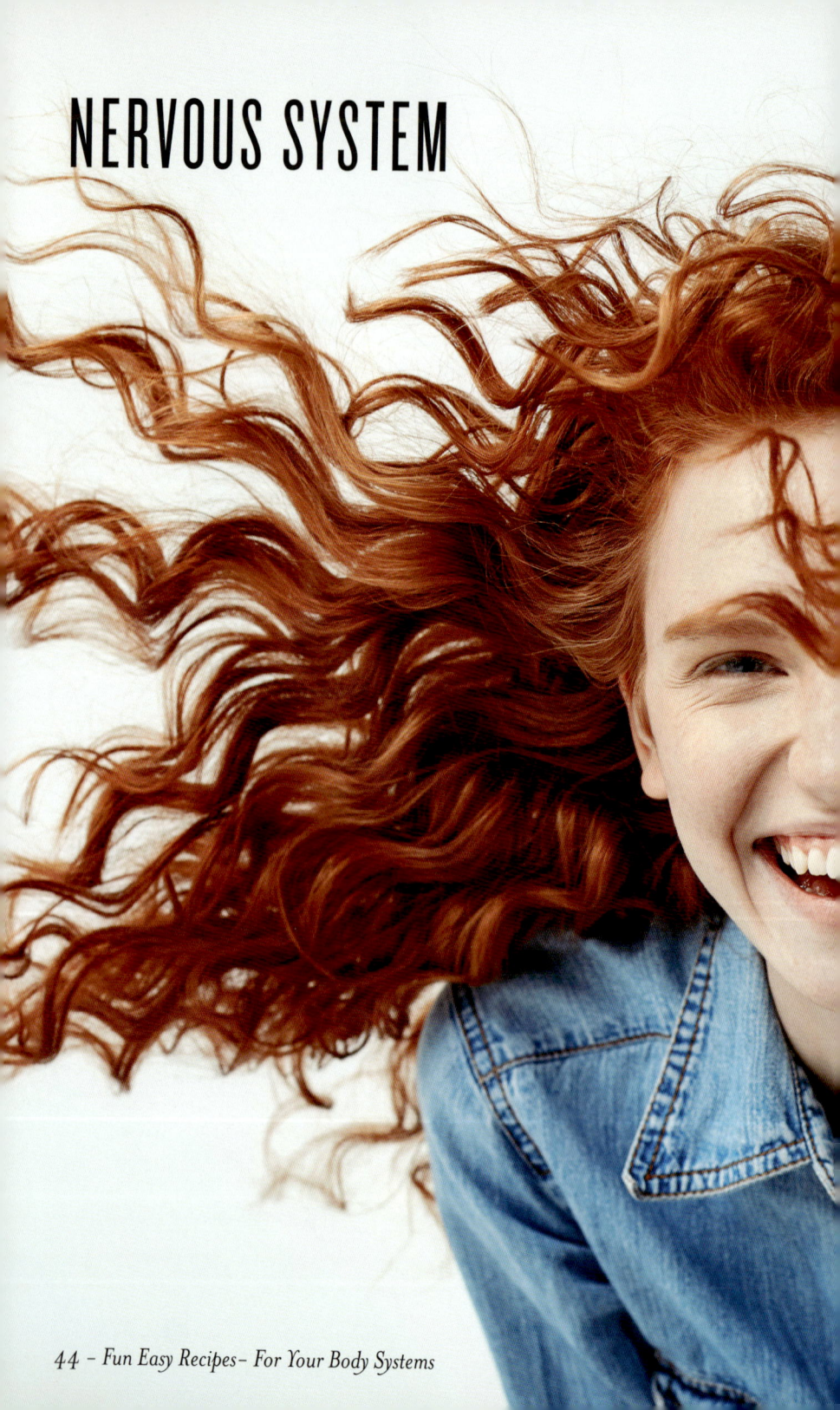

NERVOUS SYSTEM

44 - Fun Easy Recipes - For Your Body Systems

Fun Easy Recipes- For Your Body Systems - 45

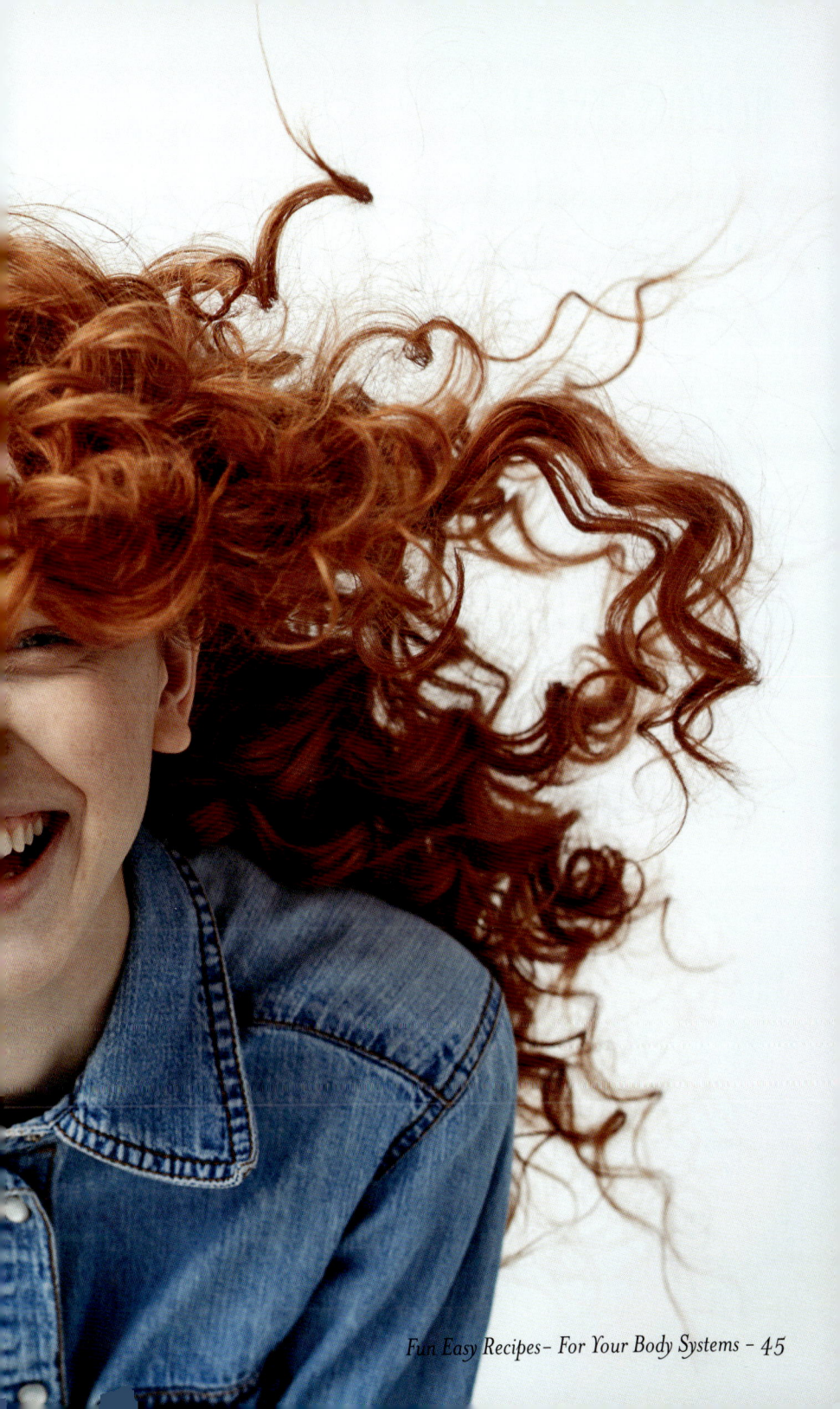

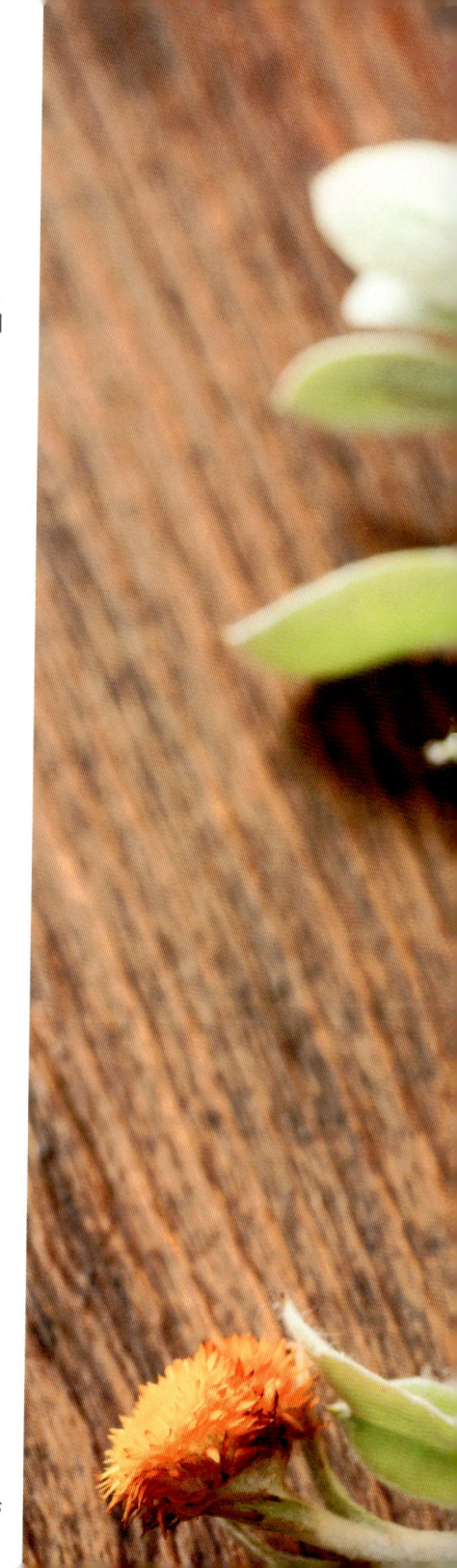

NERVOUS SYSTEM

Roll-On

Ingredients:
- 7 drops Brain Power Essential Oil
- 7 drops Helichrysum Essential Oil
- 7 drops Vetiver Essential Oil
- V-6 Vegetable Oil (or Liquid Coconut Oil)
- 10 mL Glass Roll-On Bottle

Directions:
1. Add the Essential Oils into the roll-on bottle
2. Fill with V-6 Vegetable Oil and put on the roll-on top
3. Apply onto the back of your neck to enhance concentration and focusing

Diffuser Blend

Ingredients:
- 3 drops Rosemary Essential Oil
- 3 drops Frankincense Essential Oil
- Water
- Diffuser

Directions:
1. Add water to the fill line of the diffuser
2. Put Rosemary and Frankincense Essential Oils into the water
3. Put the top of the diffuser on and press the on button
4. Breathe in to enhance concentration

Fun Easy Recipes - For Your Body Systems - 47

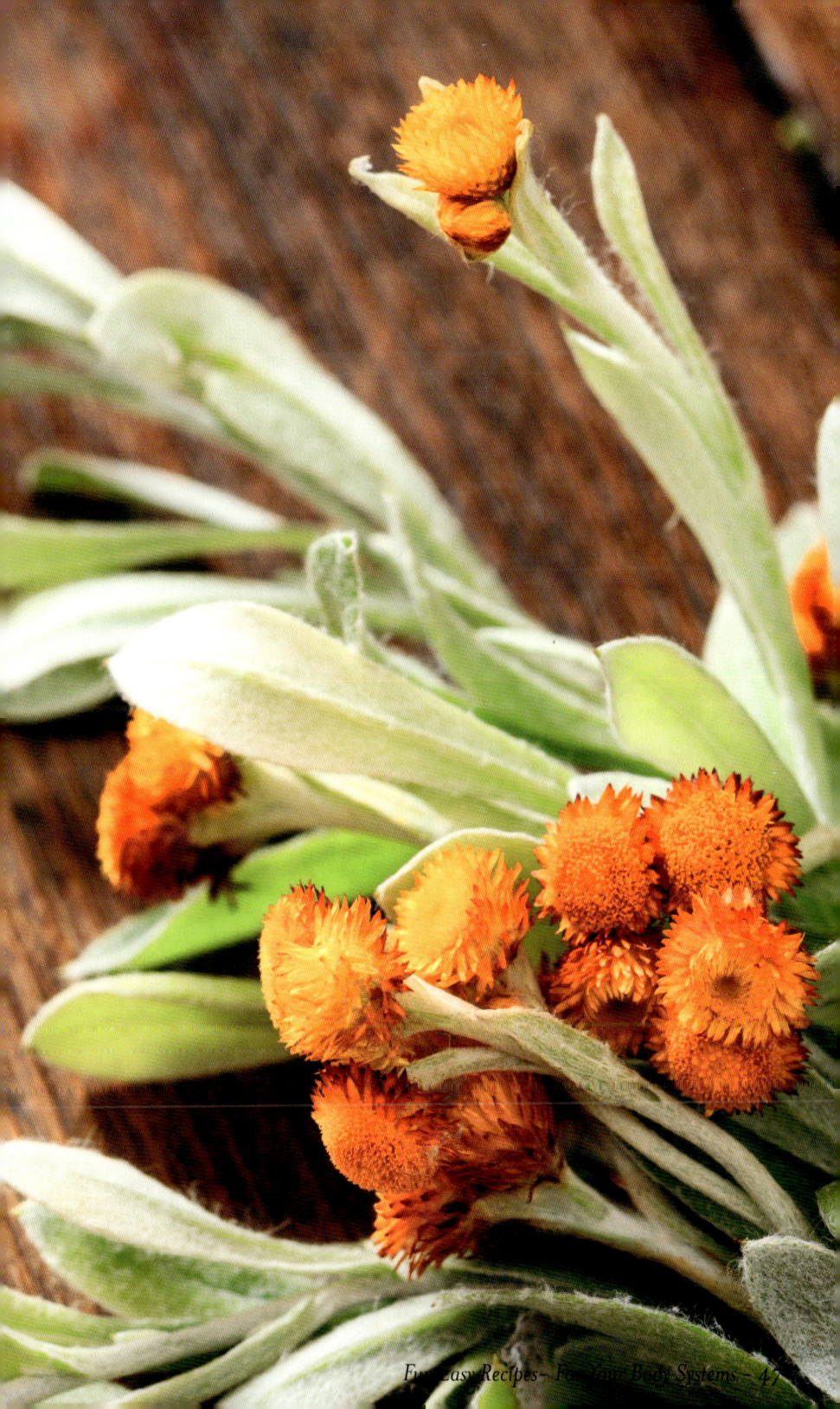

NERVOUS SYSTEM

Grounding Body Spray

Ingredients:
- 6 drops Idaho Blue Spruce Essential Oil
- 6 drops Valor Essential Oil
- Water
- 2 oz Glass Spray Bottle

Directions:
1. Add the Essential Oils into the spray bottle and fill with water. Then put on the spray bottle top.
2. Shake well before using. Spray onto your body to ground your emotions.

Happiness Spray

Ingredients:
- 5 drops Joy Essential Oil
- 7 drops Lemon Essential Oil
- Water
- 2 oz Glass Spray Bottle

Directions:
1. Add Joy and Lemon Essential Oils into the spray bottle and fill with water. Then put on the spray bottle top.
2. Shake well before using. Spray onto your body or into the air and inhale for a sense of happiness.

Fun Easy Recipes- For Your Body Systems - 49

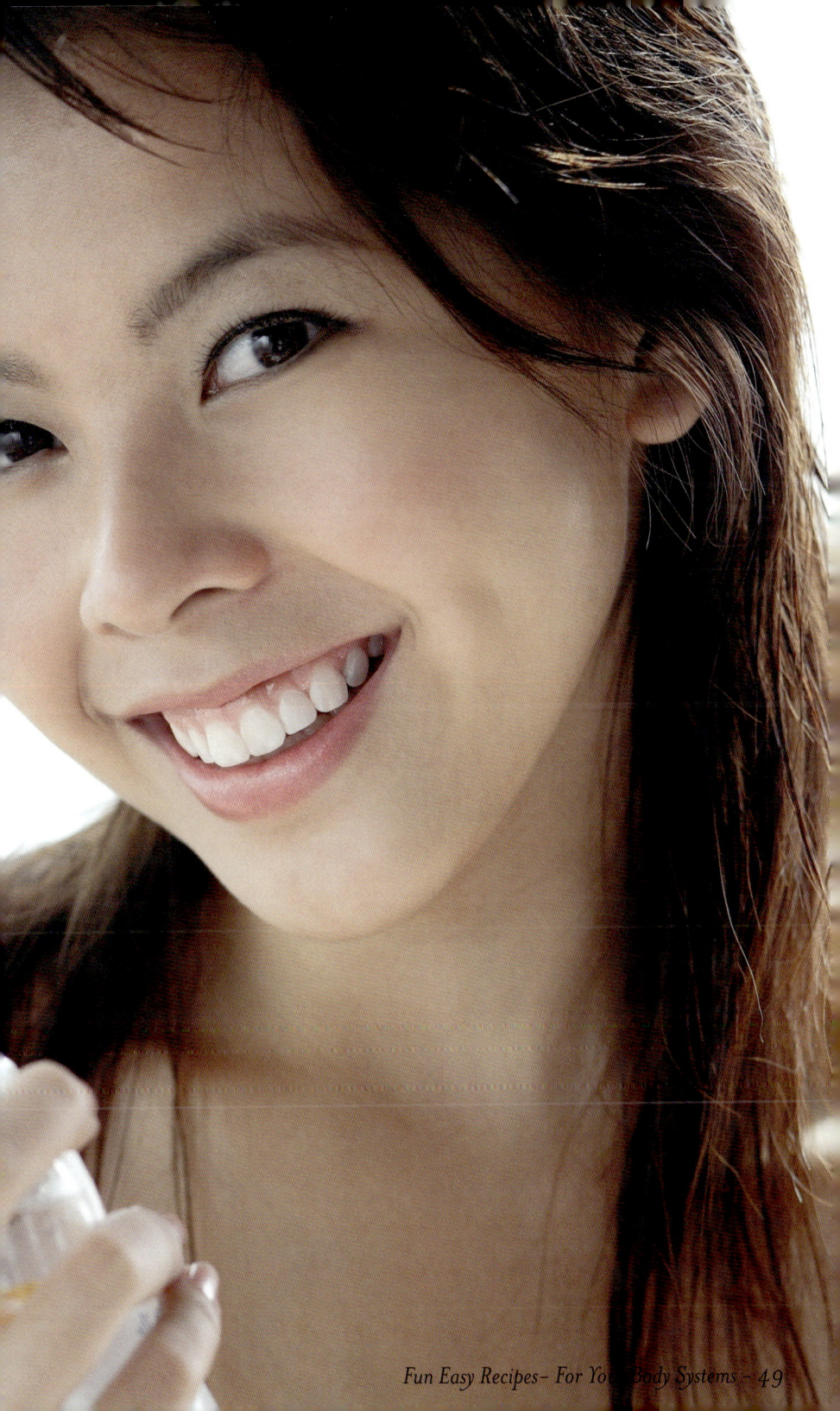

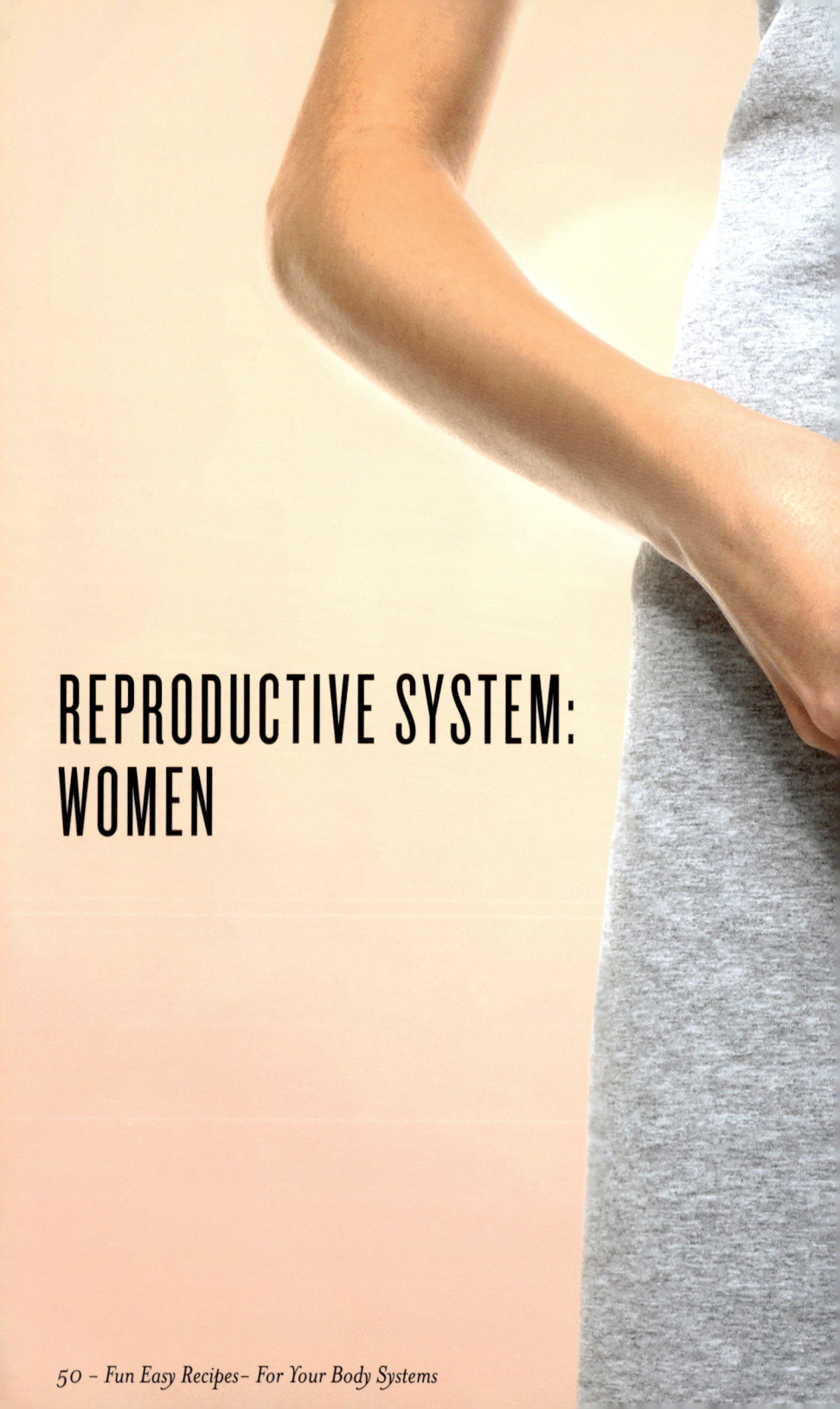

REPRODUCTIVE SYSTEM: WOMEN

50 – Fun Easy Recipes– For Your Body Systems

Fun Easy Recipes – For Your Body Systems – 51

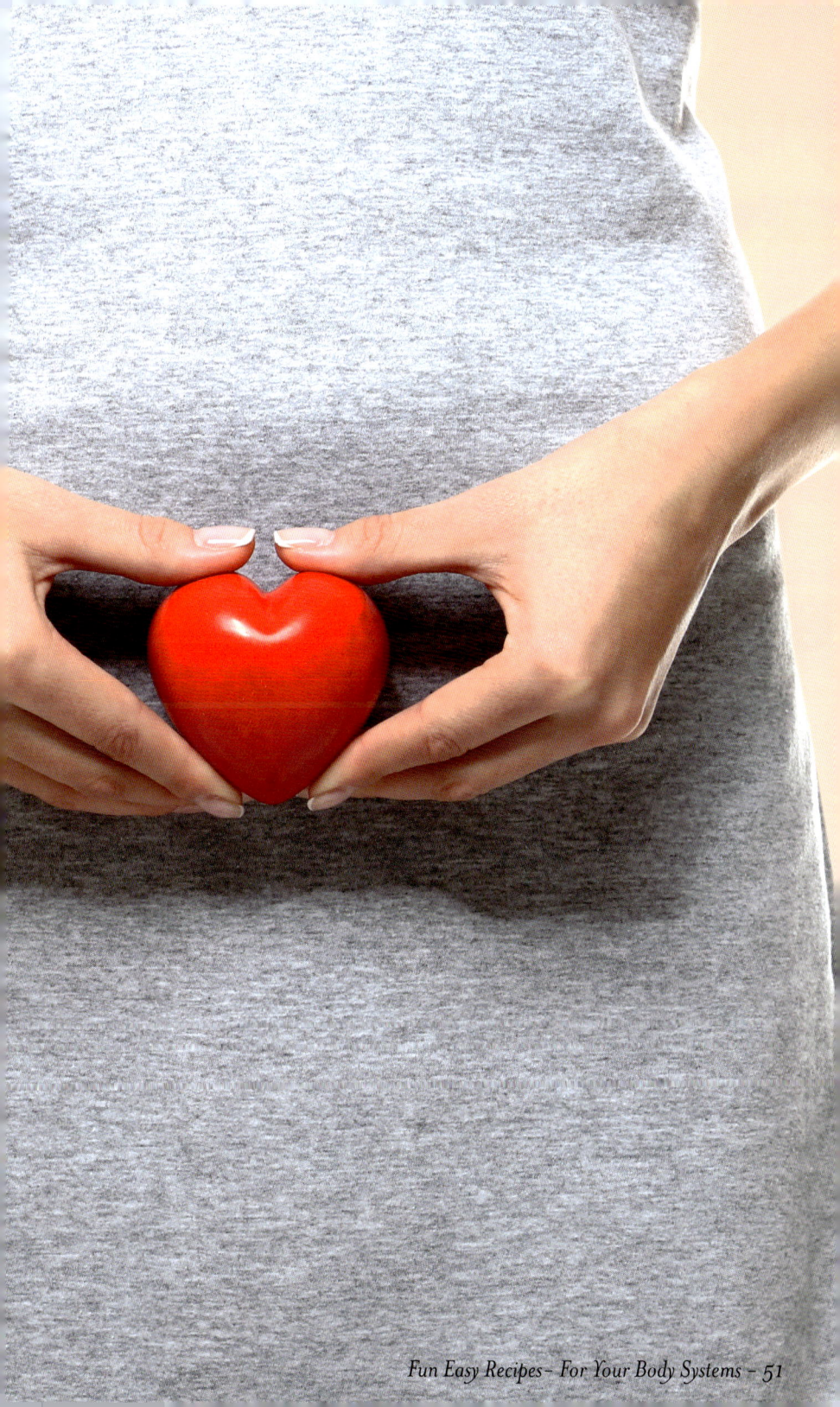

REPRODUCTIVE SYSTEM: WOMEN

Hormone Support Roll-On/Progesterone

Ingredients:
- 10 drops Progessence Plus Essential Oil
- 6 drops Stress Away Essential Oil
- V-6 Vegetable Oil (or Liquid Coconut Oil)
- 10 mL Glass Roll-On Bottle

Directions:
1. Add the Essential Oils into the roll-on bottle
2. Fill with V-6 Vegetable Oil and put on the roll-on top
3. Apply onto your wrists and neck for hormone support

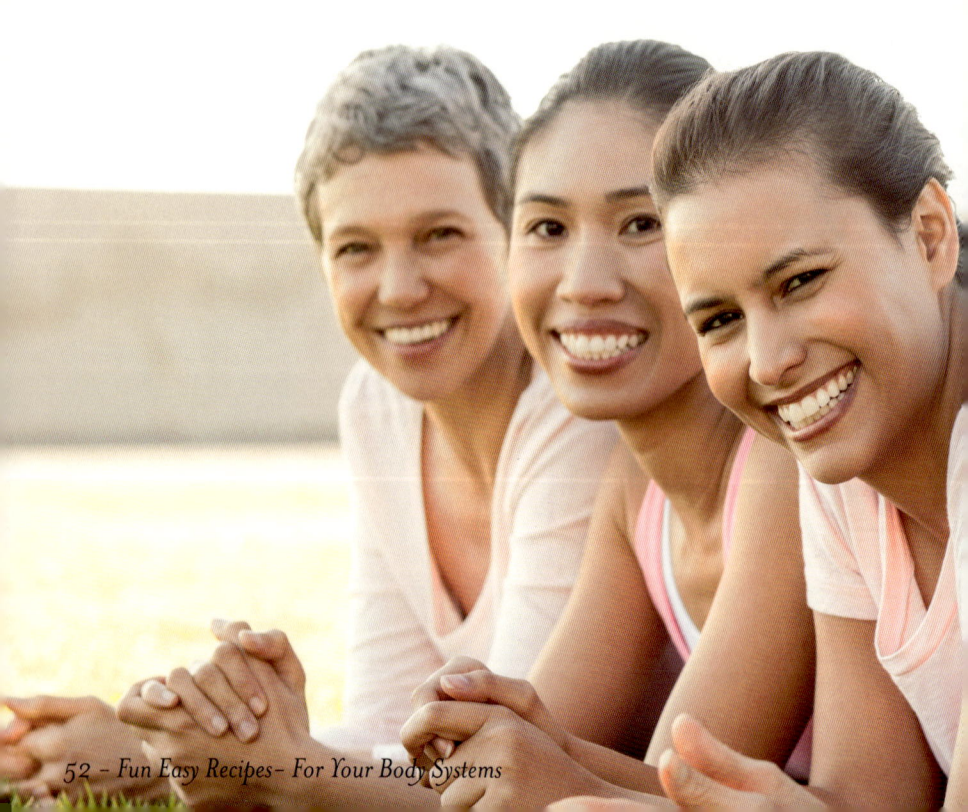

Body Spray

Ingredients:
- 6 drops Sensation Essential Oil
- 4 drops Ylang Ylang Essential Oil
- Water
- 2 oz Glass Spray Bottle

Directions:
1. Add Sensation and Ylang Ylang Essential Oils into the spray bottle
2. Fill with water and put on the spray bottle top
3. Shake well before spraying onto your body to uplift your emotions

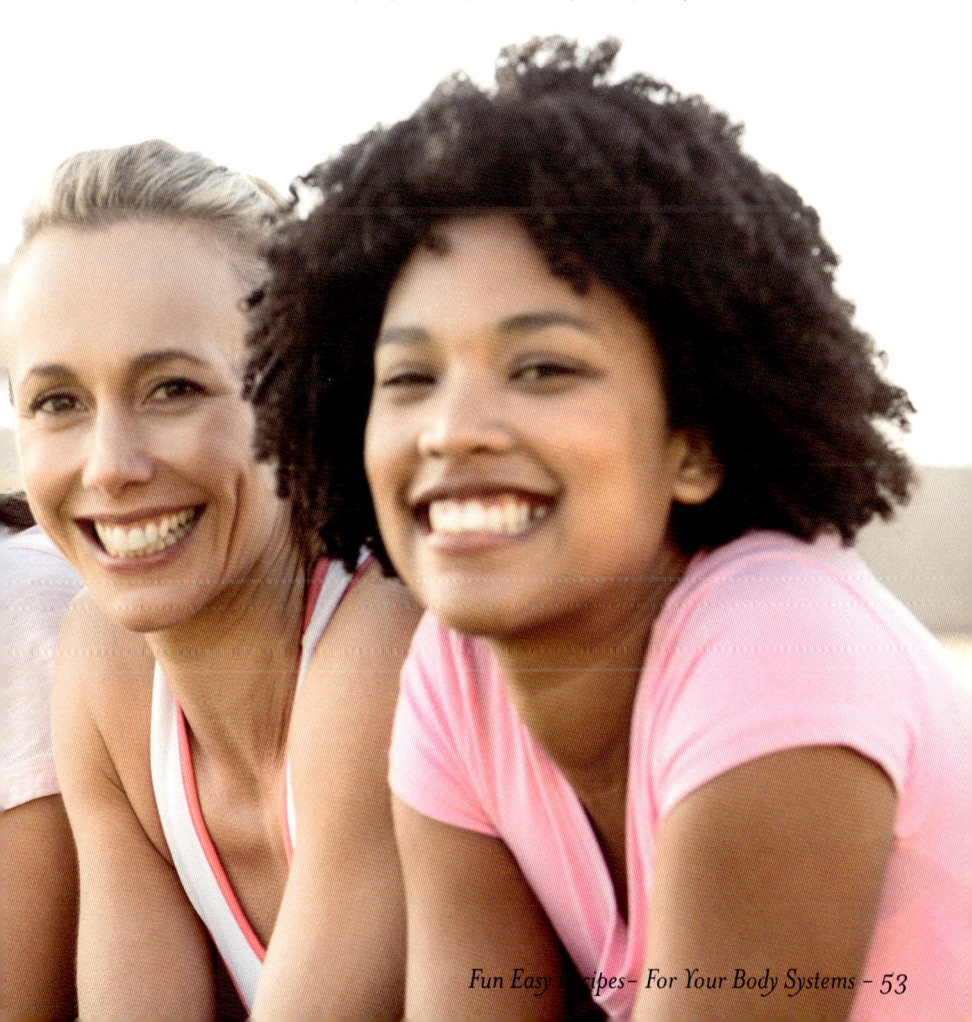

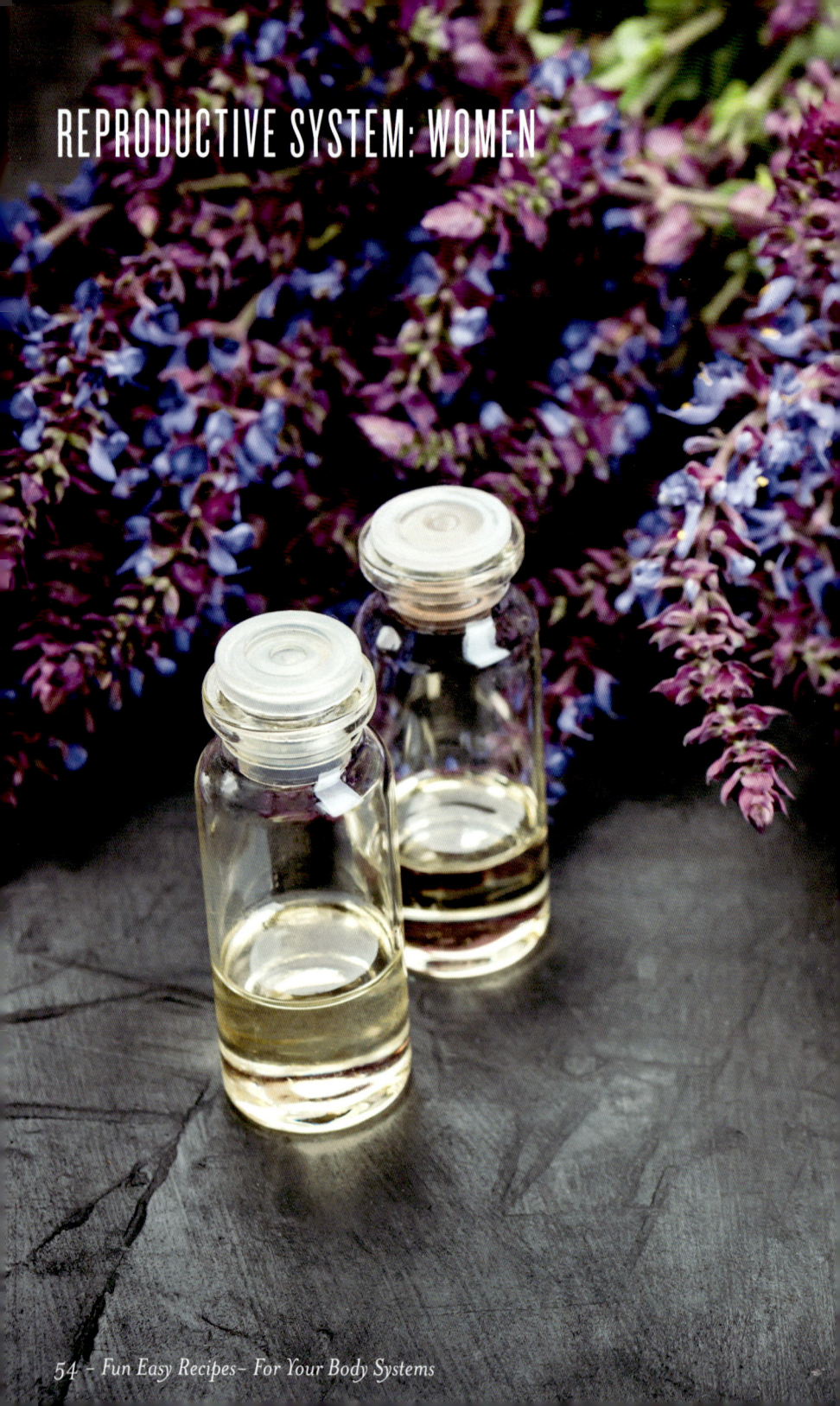

REPRODUCTIVE SYSTEM: WOMEN

Hormone Support Roll-On/Estrogen

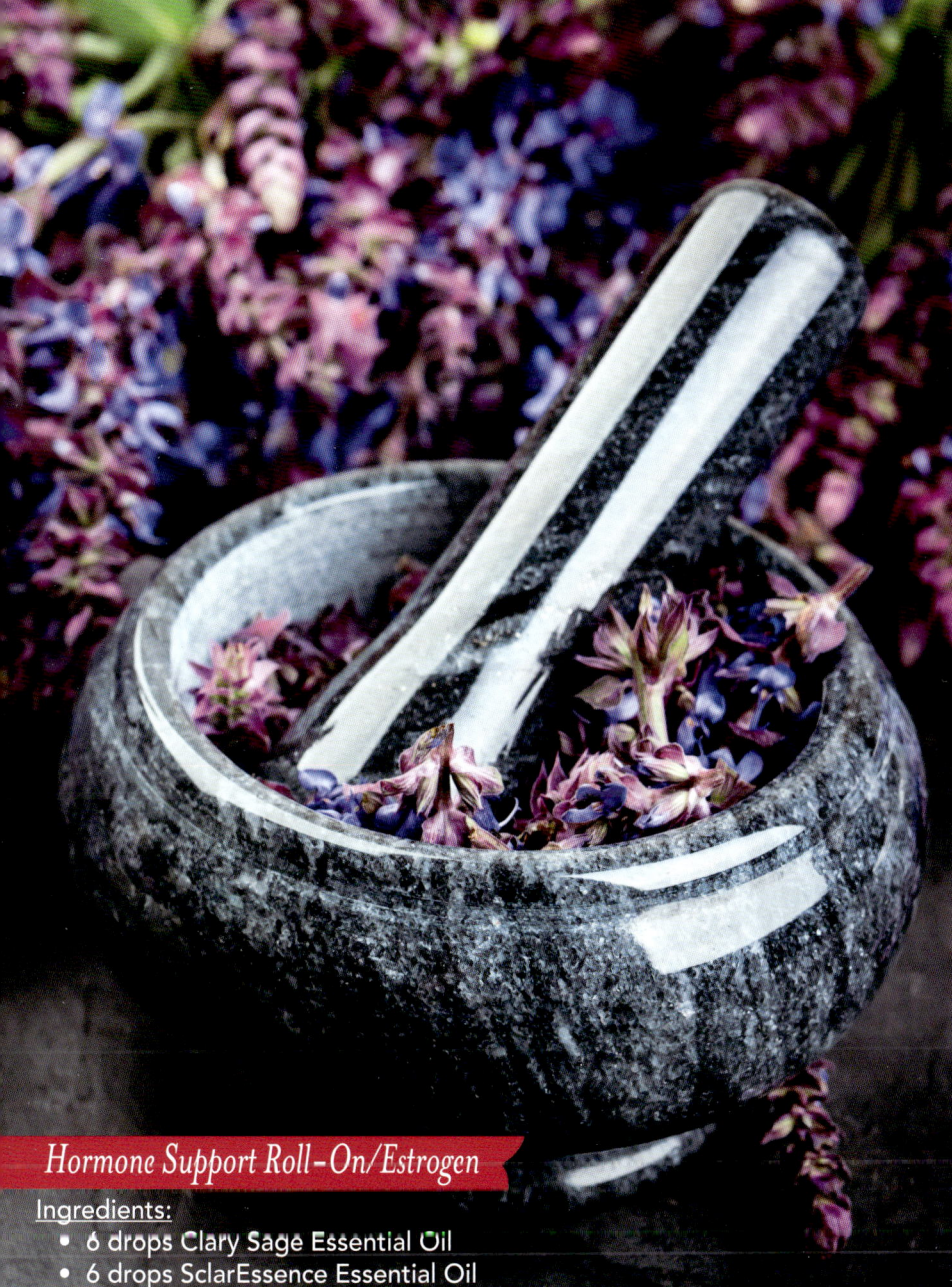

Ingredients:
- 6 drops Clary Sage Essential Oil
- 6 drops SclarEssence Essential Oil
- V-6 Vegetable Oil (or Liquid Coconut Oil)
- 10 mL Glass Roll-On Bottle

Directions:
1. Add the Essential Oils into the roll-on bottle
2. Fill with V-6 Vegetable Oil and put on the roll-on top
3. Apply onto your wrists and neck for hormone support

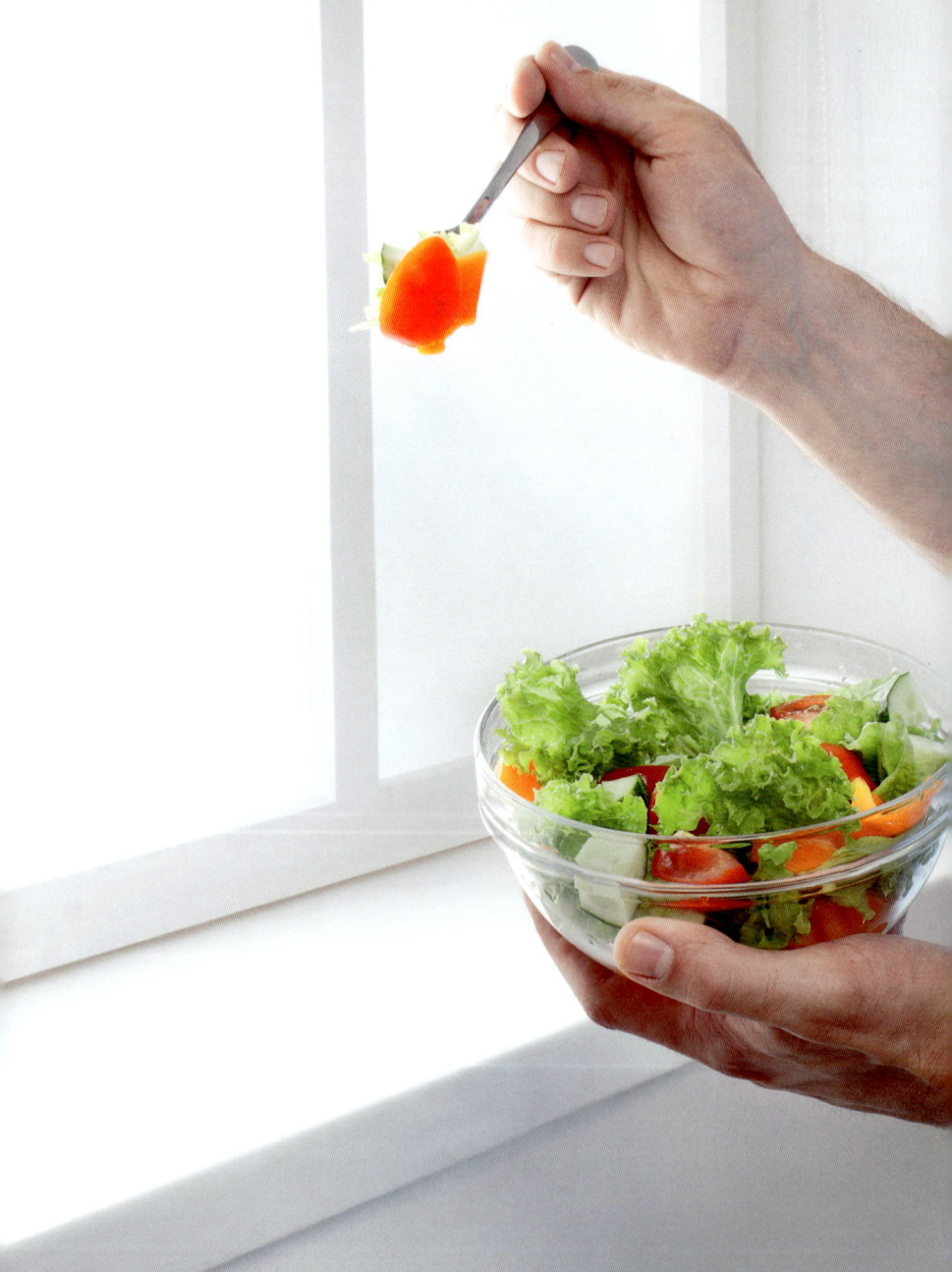

REPRODUCTIVE SYSTEM: MEN

56 - Fun Easy Recipes- For Your Body Systems

Fun Easy Recipes- For Your Body Systems - 57

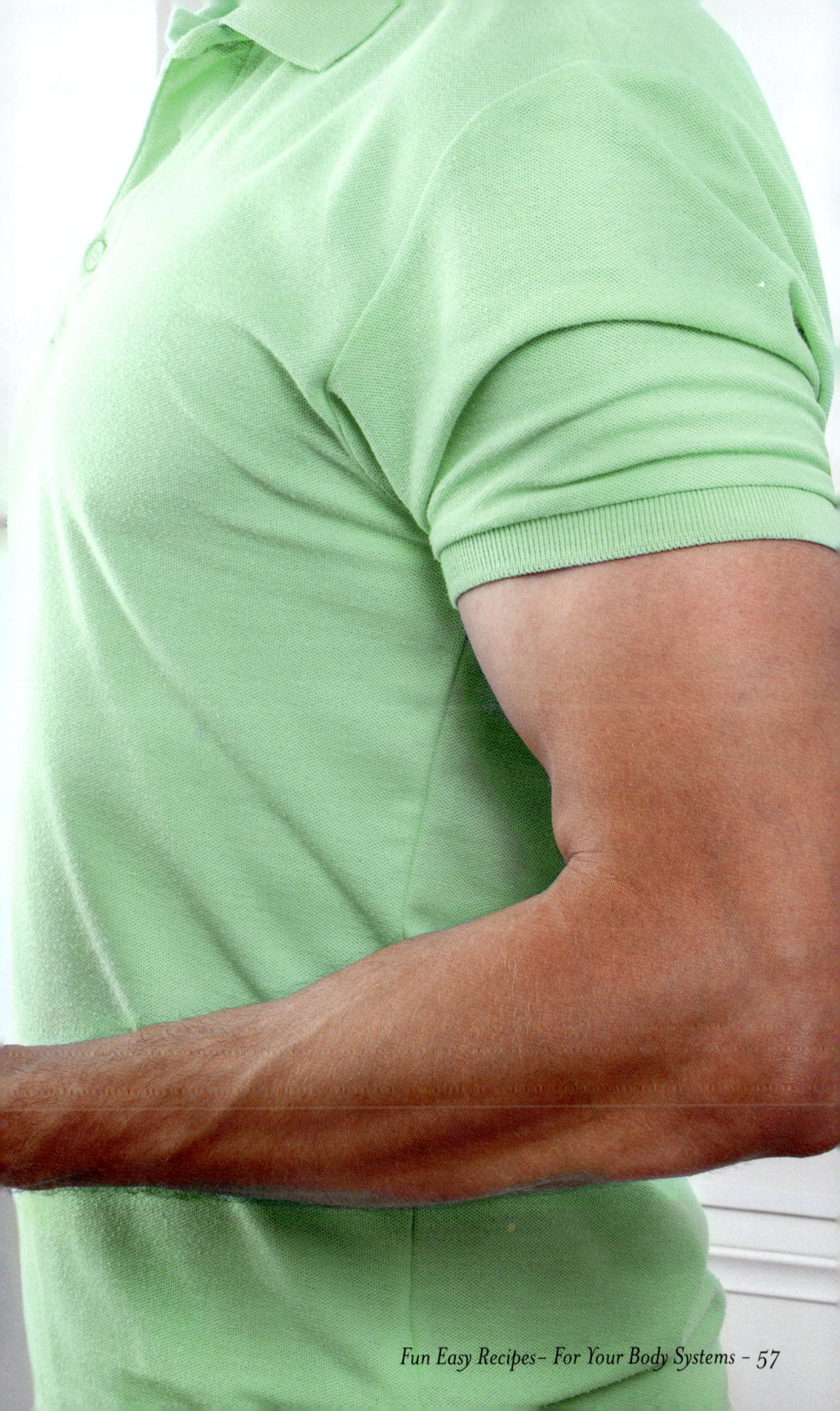

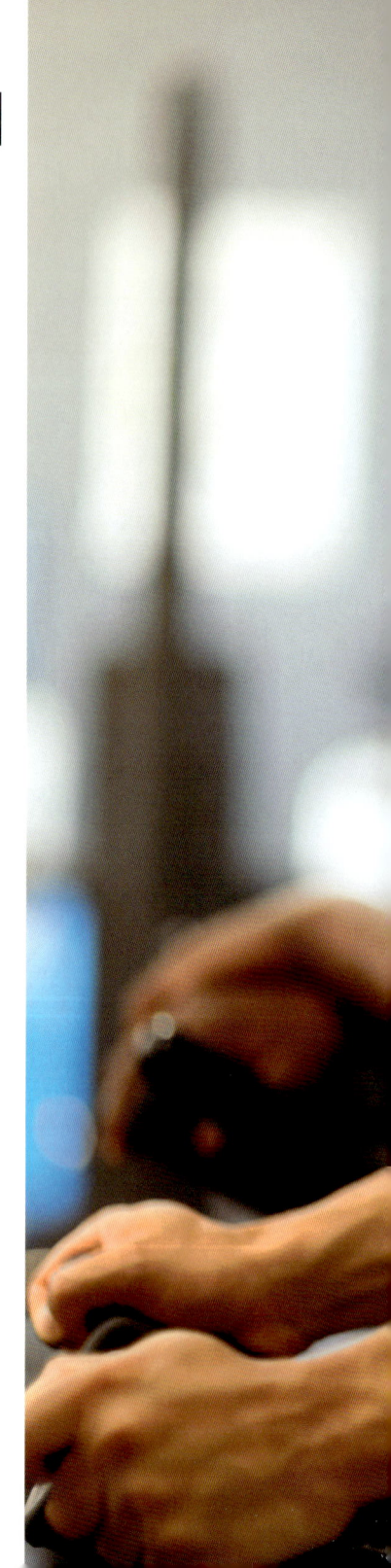

REPRODUCTIVE SYSTEM: MEN

Hormone Support Roll-On

Ingredients:
- 4 drops Mister Essential Oil
- 6 drops Shutran Essential Oil
- V-6 Vegetable Oil (or Liquid Coconut Oil)
- 10 mL Glass Roll-On Bottle

Directions:
1. Add the Essential Oils into the roll-on bottle
2. Fill with V-6 Vegetable Oil and put on the roll-on top
3. Apply onto the wrists for hormone support

Body Spray

Ingredients:
- 6 drops Northern Lights Black Spruce Essential Oil
- 6 drops Valor Essential Oil
- Water
- 2 oz Glass Spray Bottle

Directions:
1. Add the Essential Oils into the spray bottle
2. Fill with water and put on the spray bottle top
3. Shake well before spraying onto your body to uplift your emotions

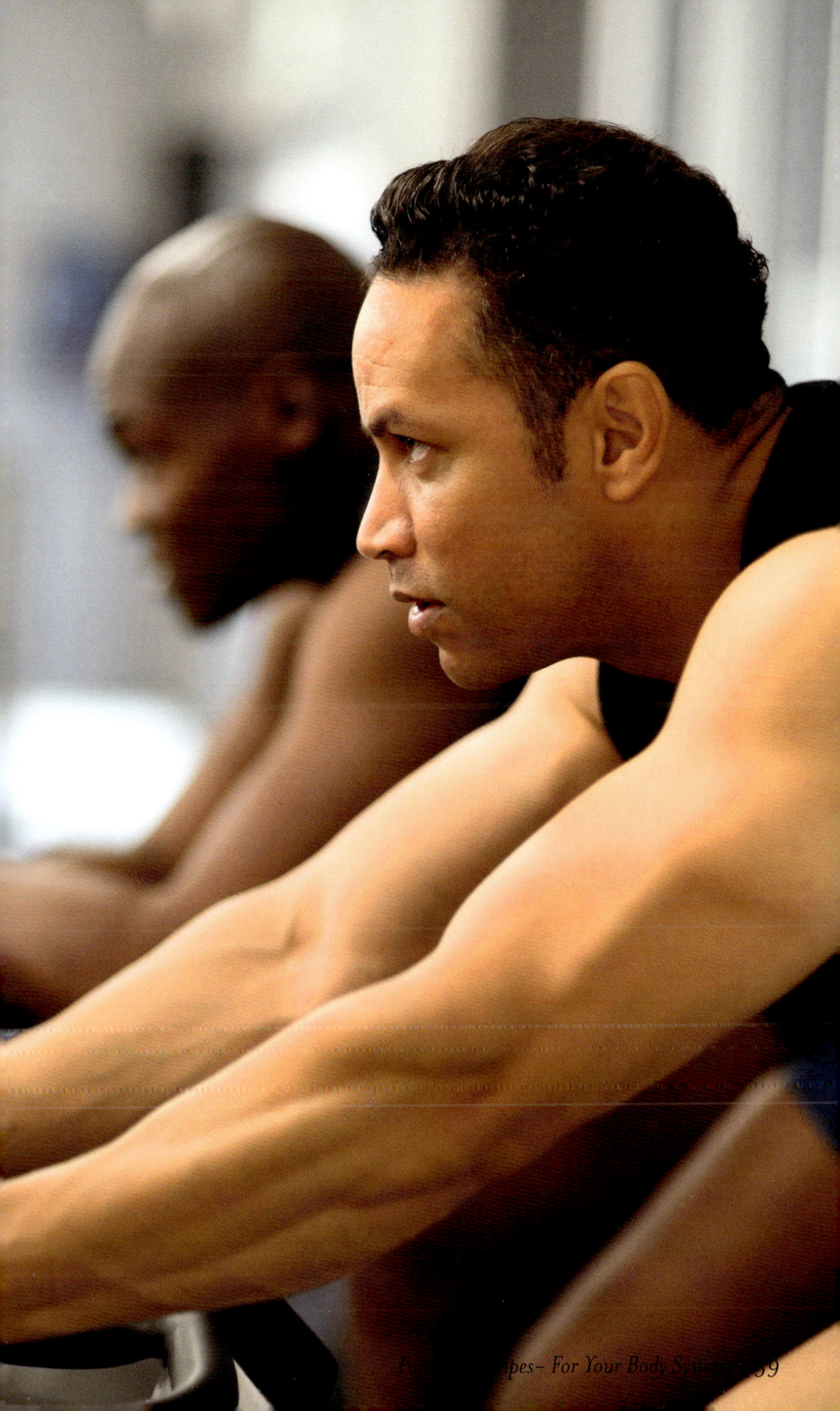

60 – *Fun Easy Recipes– For Your Body Systems*

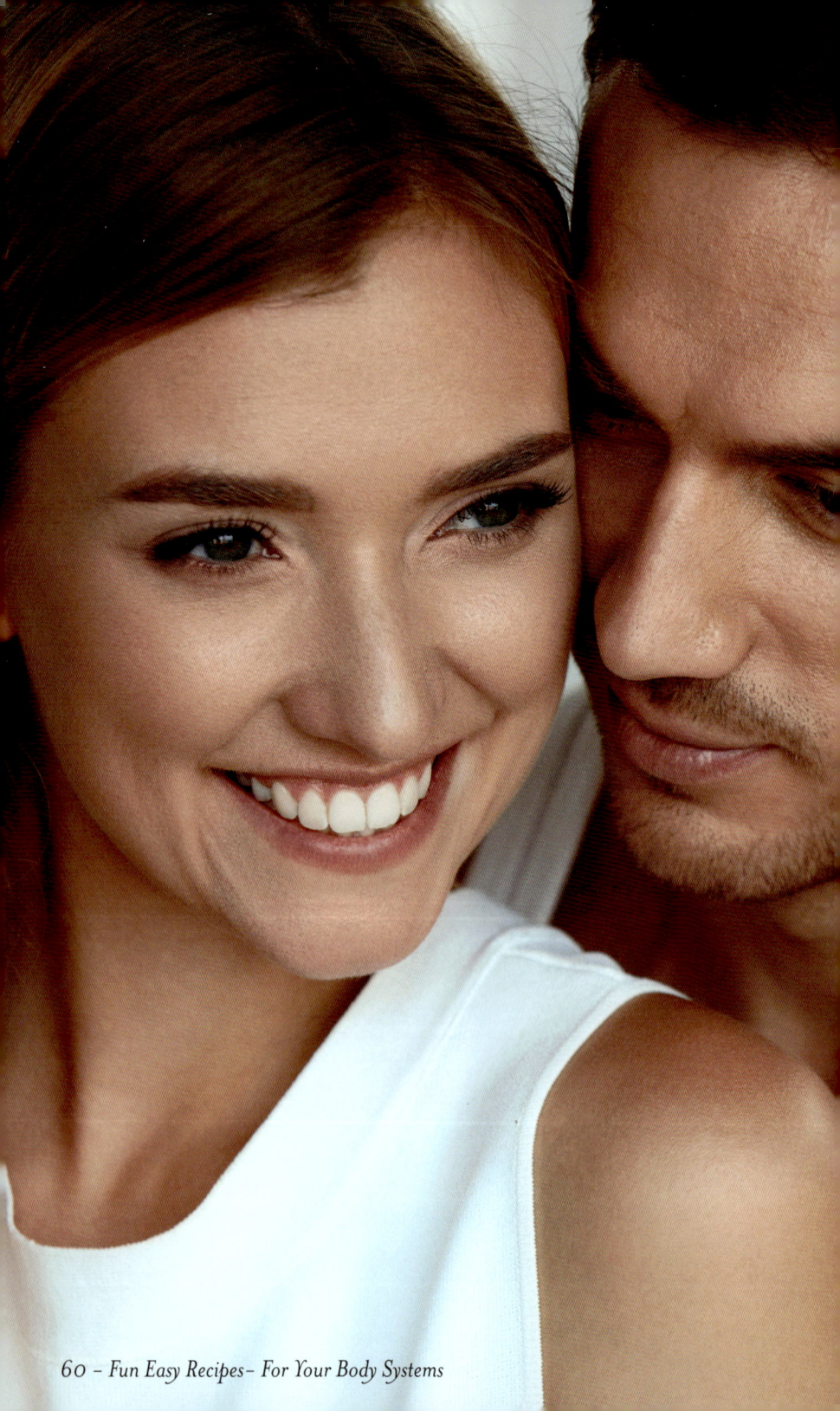

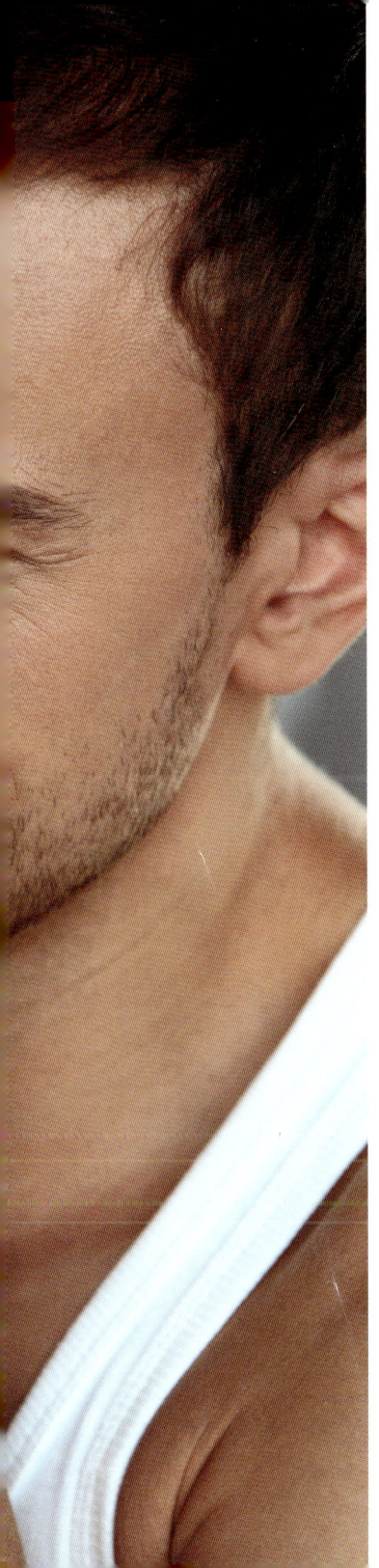

REPRODUCTIVE SYSTEM: MEN

Romance Roll-On

Ingredients:
- 10 drops Goldenrod Essential Oil
- 2 drops Mister Essential Oil
- V-6 Vegetable Oil (or Liquid Coconut Oil)
- 10 mL Glass Roll-On Bottle

Directions:
1. Add the Goldenrod and Mister Essential Oils into the roll-on bottle
2. Fill with V-6 Vegetable Oil and put on the roll-on top
3. Apply onto your wrists or inner thighs as needed

RESPIRATORY SYSTEM

Fun Easy Recipes- For Your Body Systems - 63

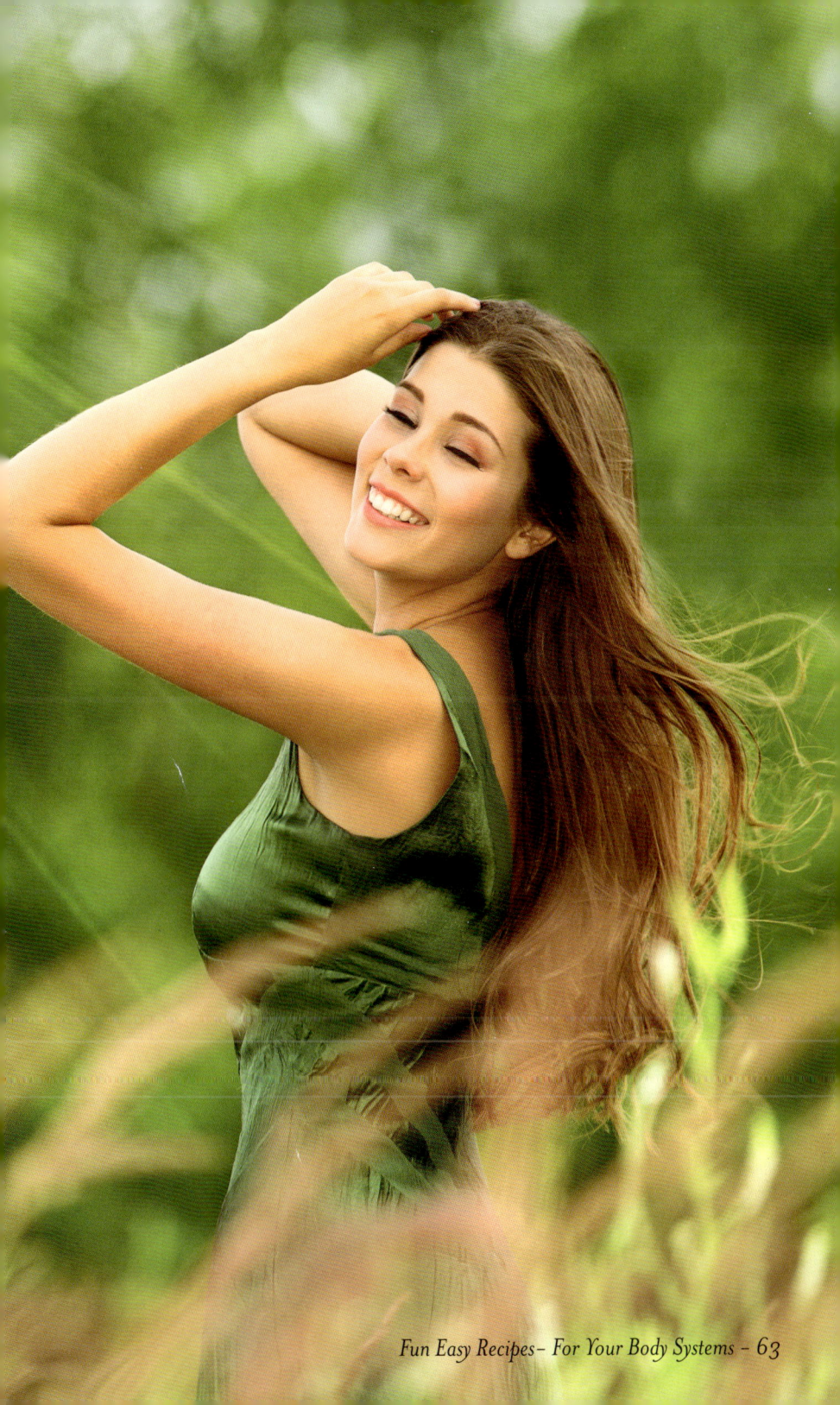

RESPIRATORY SYSTEM

Diffuser Blend

Ingredients:
- 3 drops R.C. Essential Oil
- 3 drops Raven Essential Oil
- Water
- Diffuser

Directions:
1. Add water to the fill line of the diffuser
2. Put R.C. and Raven Essential Oils into the water
3. Put the top of the diffuser on and press the on button
4. Breathe in to support your respiratory system

Roll-On

Ingredients:
- 7 drops Eucalyptus Radiata Essential Oil
- 7 drops Ravintsara Essential Oil
- V-6 Vegetable Oil (or Liquid Coconut Oil)
- 10 mL Glass Roll-On Bottle

Directions:
1. Add the Essential Oils into the roll-on bottle
2. Fill with V-6 Vegetable Oil and put on the roll-on top
3. Apply onto your chest to support the respiratory system

Fun Easy Recipes– For Your Body Systems – 65

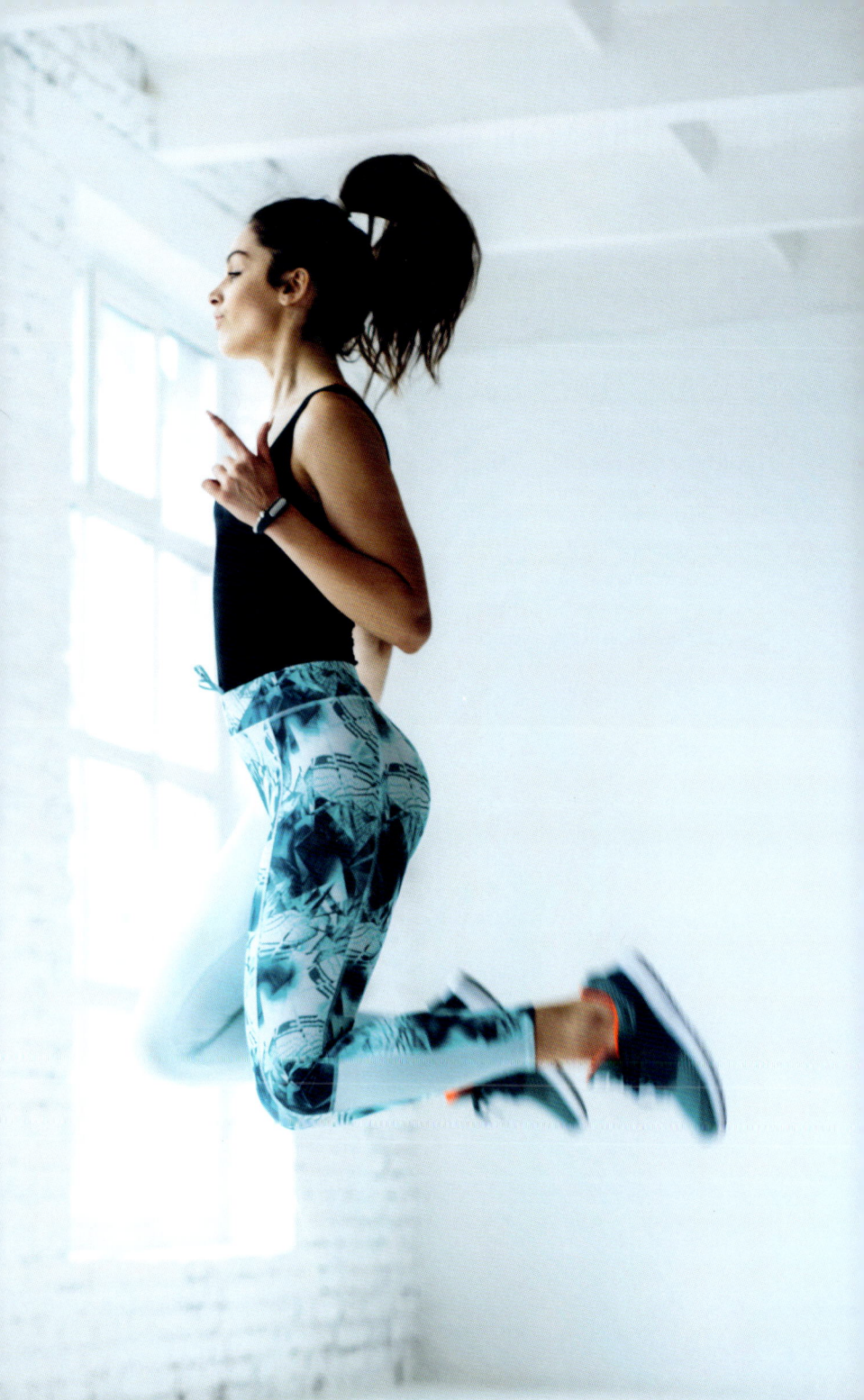

RESPIRATORY SYSTEM

Body Rub

Ingredients:
- 3 drops Dorado Azul Essential Oil
- 6 drops Raven Essential Oil
- 1/3 cup Virgin Coconut Oil
- 4 oz Glass Mason Jar

Directions:
1. Add the Coconut Oil, Dorado Azul and Raven Essential Oils into a glass bowl
2. Mix the ingredients together
3. Place the mixture into the jar. Apply a small amount onto your chest for respiratory support

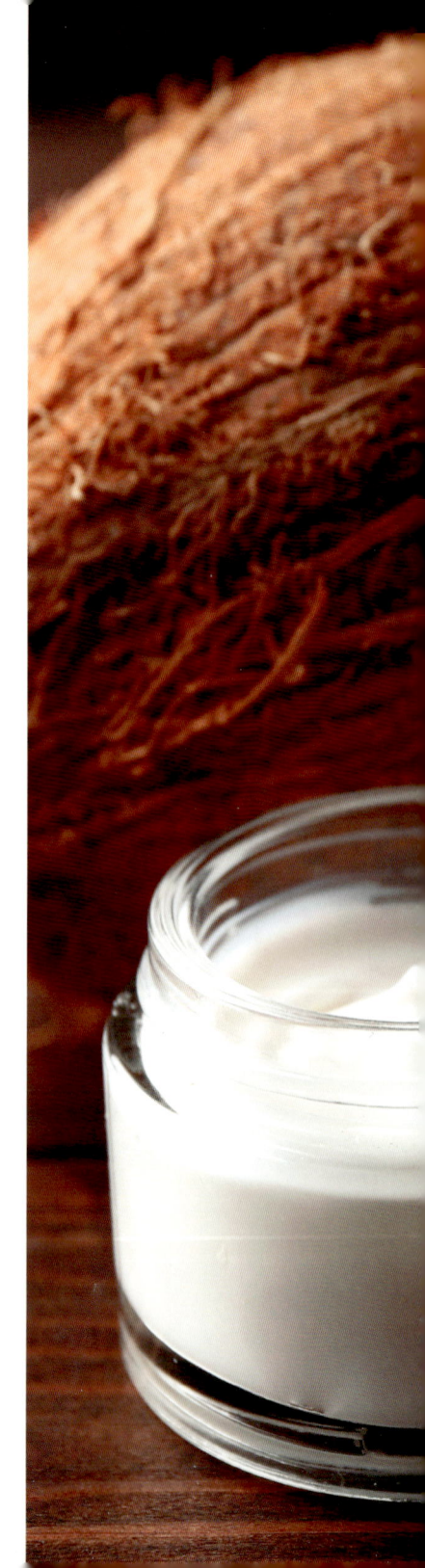

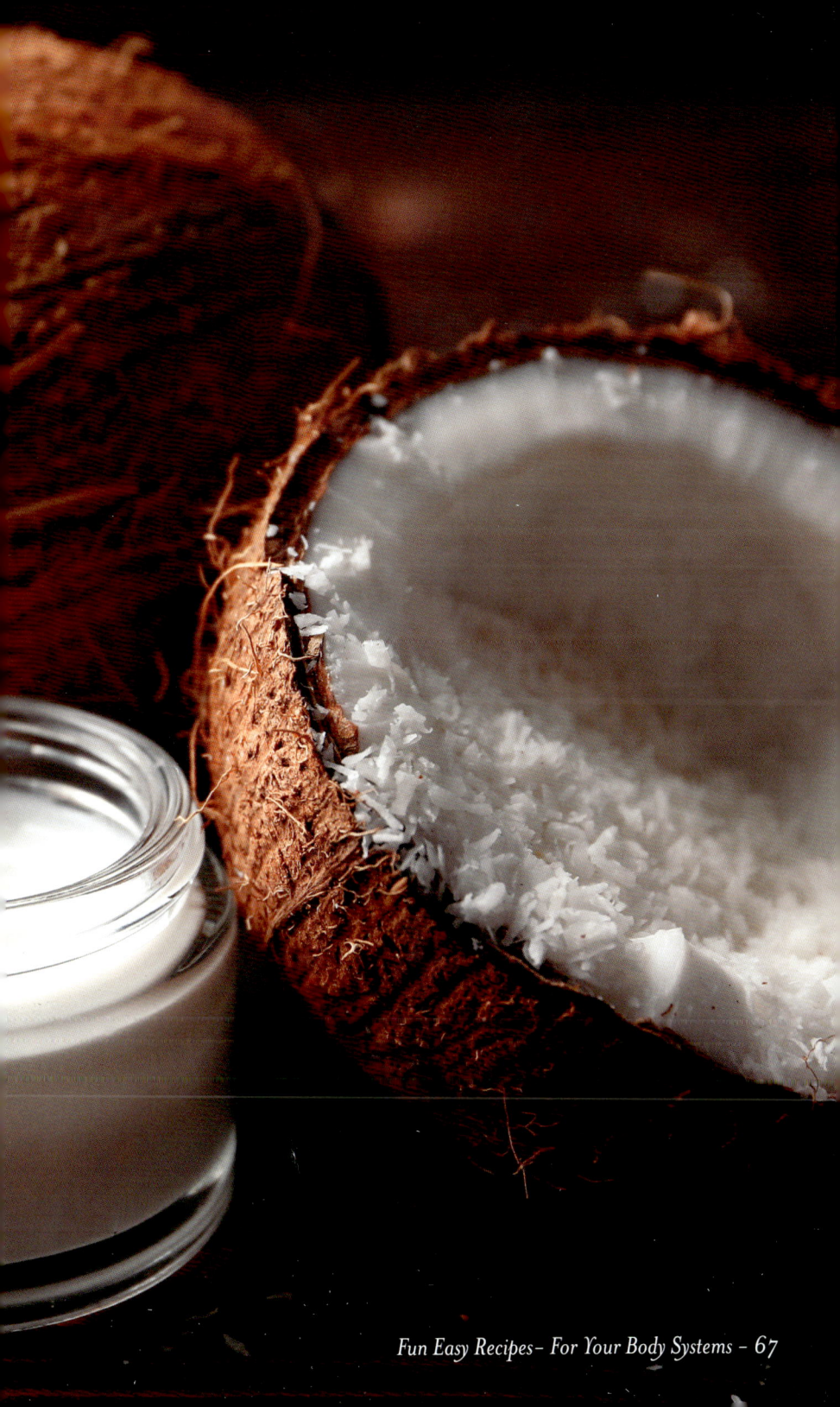

URINARY SYSTEM

Fun Easy Recipes- For Your Body Systems - 69

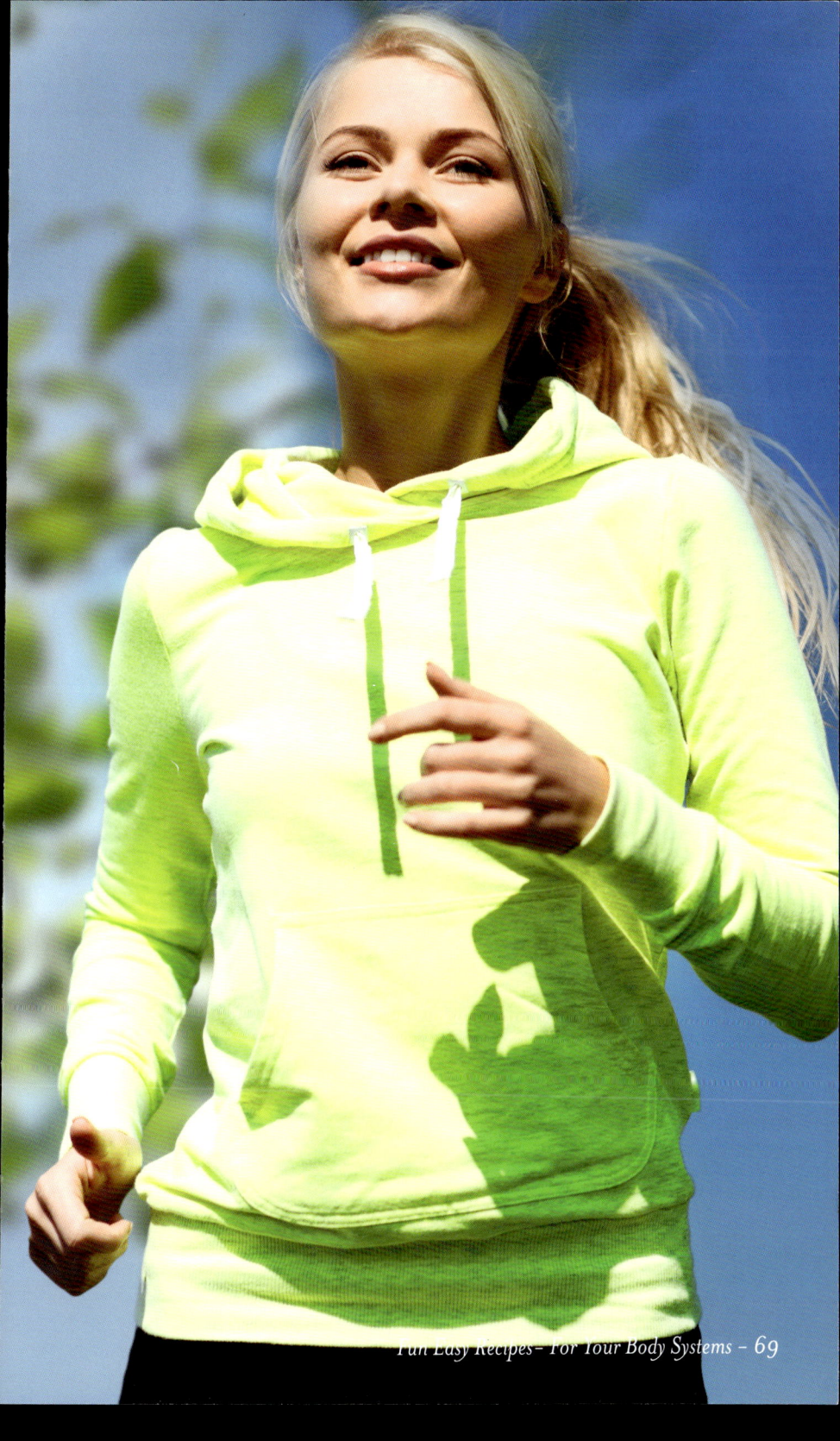

URINARY SYSTEM

Roll-On

Ingredients:
- 10 drops Juniper Essential Oil
- 8 drops Cypress Essential Oil
- V-6 Vegetable Oil (or Liquid Coconut Oil)
- 10 mL Glass Roll-On Bottle

Directions:
1. Add the Essential Oils into the roll-on bottle
2. Fill with V-6 Vegetable Oil and put on the roll-on top
3. Apply onto your lower abdomen and kidney area to support the urinary system

Capsule

Ingredients:
- 6 drops Thieves Vitality Essential Oil
- 4 drops Thyme Vitality Essential Oil
- Vegetable Capsule

Directions:
1. Add the Thieves Vitality and Thyme Vitality Essential Oils into the capsule
2. Ingest one capsule for urinary support as needed

Fun Easy Recipes– For Your Body Systems - 71

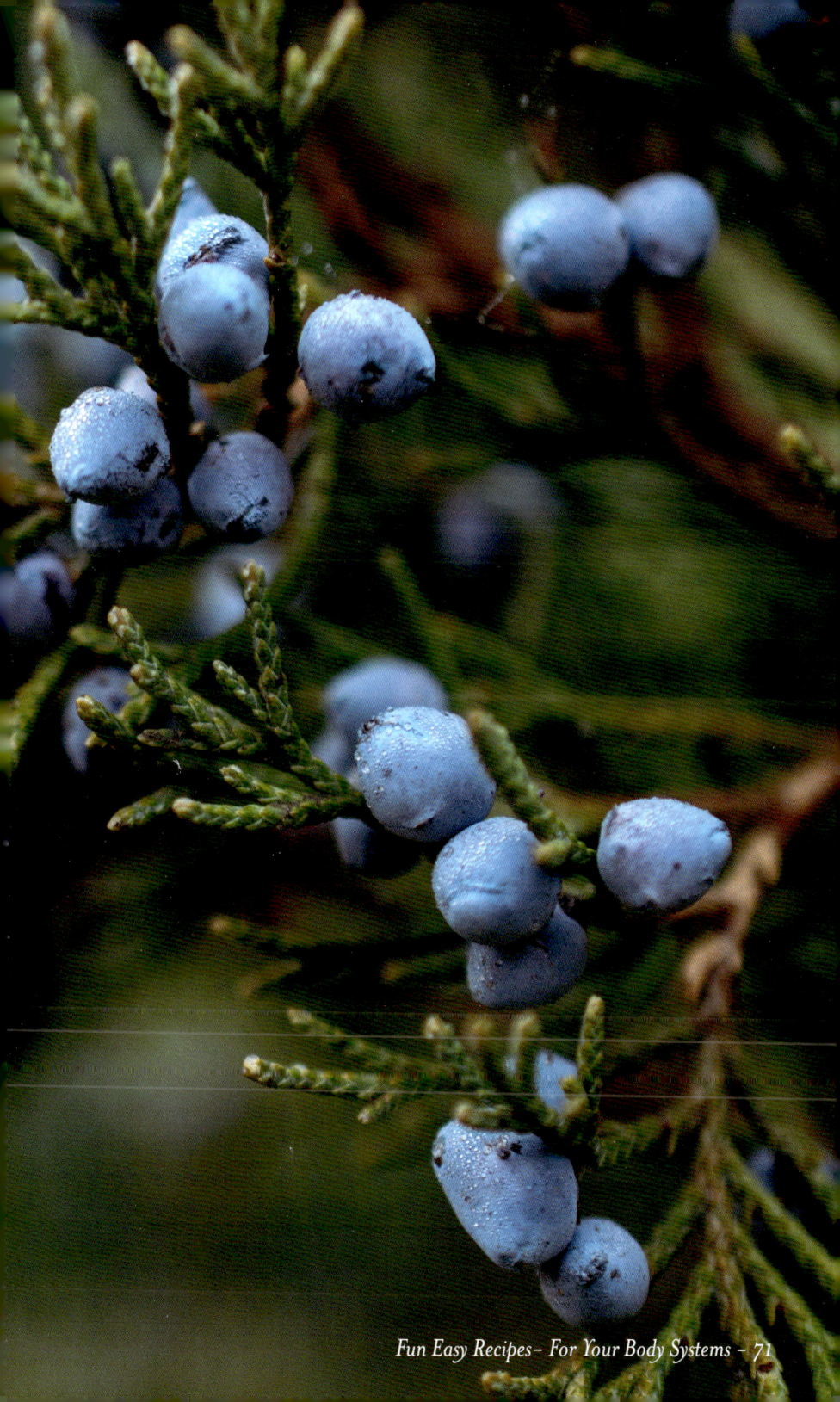

URINARY SYSTEM

Kid's Nighttime Support Roll-On

Ingredients:
- 10 drops Cypress Essential Oil
- 5 drops Valor Essential Oil
- 5 drops Peace & Calming Essential Oil
- V-6 Vegetable Oil (or Liquid Coconut Oil)
- 10 mL Glass Roll-On Bottle

Directions:
1. Add the Essential Oils into the roll-on bottle
2. Fill with V-6 Vegetable Oil and put on the roll-on top
3. Apply onto the lower abdomen to support the urinary system overnight

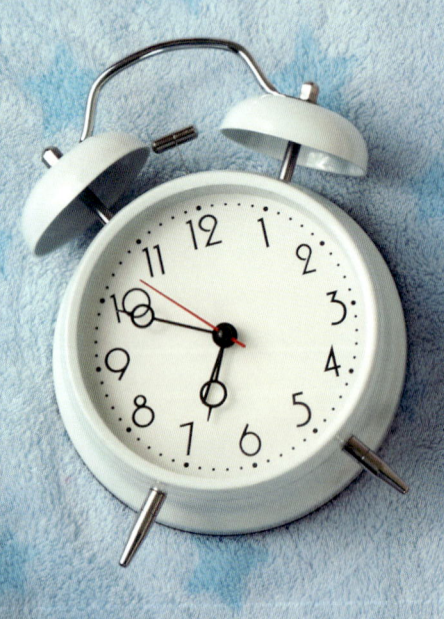

For Your Body Systems – 73

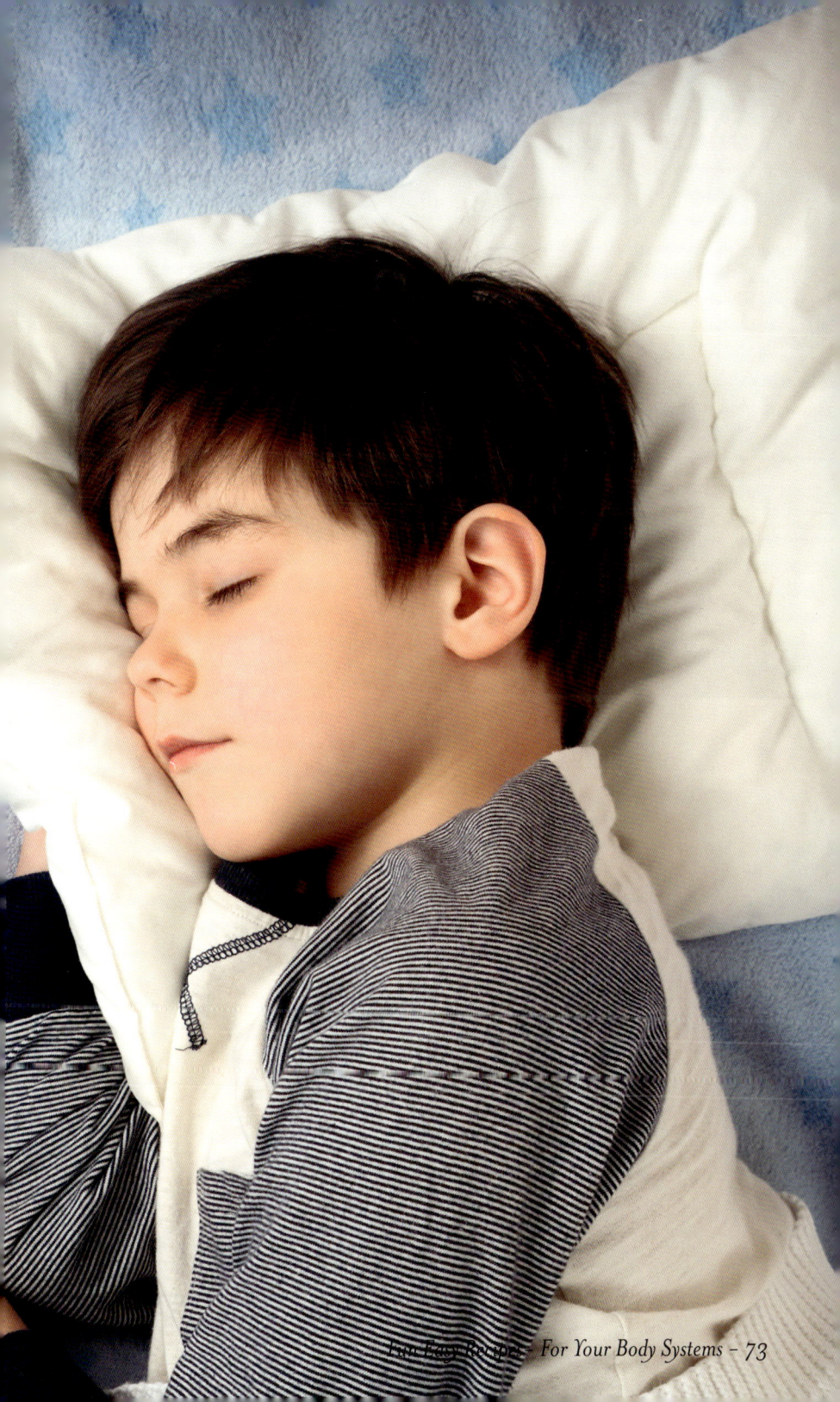

ESSENTIAL REWARDS

Save Money ~ Transfer Buy ~ Get Rewarded

- Receive 10-25% back in product credit EVERY MONTH and it's cumulative

- Redeem the points for FREE PRODUCTS!

- Receive Flat Rate and Reduced Shipping

- FREE GIFTS for members that stay on Essential Rewards for 3, 6, 9, and 12 months!

- Purchase your Healthy Lifestyle products through Young Living (ex: toothpaste, deodorant, shampoo, body wash, etc.)

- ONLY Requirement: place a 50 PV order each month

10% 1-3 MONTHS   **20%** 4-24 MONTHS   **25%** 25+ MONTHS

GIFTS AT 3, 6, AND 9 MONTHS   **SPECIAL GIFT** AT 12 MONTHS
Exclusive Essential Oil Blend "Loyalty"

74 - Fun Easy Recipes- For Your Body Systems

By the same authors:

FUN EASY RECIPES

With Your Starter Kit from Young Living

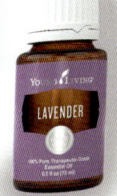

Dive into your starter kit with over 40 easy recipes

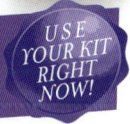

USE YOUR KIT RIGHT NOW!

Chelsa Bruno & Dana Ripepe

Buy and share *Fun Easy Recipes* — the premiere volume including fabulous recipes designed to help you make use of your Young Living Starter Kit!